The Health Habit:

27 Small Daily Changes for Physical Energy, Mental Peace, and Peak Performance

by Nick Trenton

www.NickTrenton.com

Table of Contents

Introduction

I'm going to tell you a story you've never heard before but which is probably painfully familiar to you. Mr. X is a fat slob who desperately wants to get healthy, get fit, and feel something he hasn't felt in ages—pride in his appearance. Mr. X, despite being a fat slob, is actually an expert on diets . . . after all, he's tried every diet out there. And nobody starts a new exercise regime with as much zeal and dedication as Mr. X.

But then again, nobody quits as often as he does, either. All Mr. X's grand plans seem to crumble after a few days or weeks. Somehow, nothing sticks. He loses and gains the same twenty pounds over and over again. It's not that he doesn't want to be better—he wants it more than anything in the world. But the truth is that he simply isn't going about things in the right way.

Long story short, Mr. X *did* finally find his way in the end. He realized he had to unlearn much of what he thought he knew, get honest with himself, and work hard in a way he hadn't known to work before. If you haven't guessed it yet, Mr. X in this story is *me*.

Here's a question for you: is real change possible?

Is it possible for people to completely transform their bodies, their minds, and their behaviors?

If you've picked up this book, you might on one hand sincerely *wish* for genuine change . . . but on the other hand, doubt that it's really possible for you. If you've ever tried a diet and failed with it a few days later, or committed to a new exercise regime only to give it up within a month, then this book was written for you.

Change is not easy, no, but it is absolutely one hundred percent possible—yes, for *you*. This book is a condensed manual containing the key principles that are needed for any successful lifestyle change, whether your goal is to lose a few pounds and look better, or to completely overhaul your way of life, from diet to exercise to daily habits.

You already know that you want to change. That you have to change. This book will show you *how* to change. Unfortunately, good intentions are seldom enough. You need a clear, effective strategy for charting the path from where you are now to where you want to be.

In the chapters that follow, you will learn how to make *lasting changes* to your life one habit at a time. You'll learn how to dig deep into your values and principles so they can inspire workable goals that you can then proactively transform into action. You'll learn the power of cumulative effort and habit, why dedication and commitment are so important, and how to pre-empt and outsmart those inevitable setbacks. After reading this book, those setbacks will no longer have the same power to derail you. Big dreams are made of small actions—and this book is all about how to begin, right now, to start walking that path that leads directly to the place you want to go.

At this point, you probably don't need to be told how important it is to avoid junk food, or to drink water instead of soda. You already *know* that you need to be exercising, to be sleeping well, to be managing stress. This book has nothing to add in that area. Unlike other health and wellness manuals, this book is about the HOW, the real nuts and bolts of what to do day in and day out to make sure you become a person who automatically avoids junk food, drinks water, and exercises.

As you read some of the advice below, it will likely seem . . . humble. But remember, big dreams are made of small actions. Consistency, commitment, and having the intelligence to preempt and avoid pitfalls are all that's needed. These techniques are free and available to anyone. Don't let their simplicity fool you, though: every single person out there who has drastically changed their lives for the better has, in some way or another, used the very techniques described in this book. And you could soon be one of them.

If you're feeling doubtful right now, that's okay. It would be weird if you weren't! But I know the techniques I'm going to outline in the following chapters do work, even though they're deceptively simple. I know this because they worked for me. I've seen them work for others time and again.

Let's change the question. Let's not ask, "Is real change possible?" but ask instead, "**How** do I make real change?" Everything I've learned tells me there is only one answer: one step at a time.

Intelligence to preempt and avoid pitfalls

Chapter 1: Morning Routine

Choosing the Kind of Routine You Should Have in the Morning

Let's start with the first step, then. Not all morning routines are created equal. There is no one-size-fits-all and no cheat code when it comes to creating any useful habit in life! It's no use looking to inspirational figures or admired celebrities and asking what they do every morning. If it doesn't work for *your* life, then it doesn't work, period. So, if you read somewhere that Benjamin Franklin used to get up at 4 o'clock every morning, that doesn't mean that diligently setting your alarm for that time will bring you any closer to a healthier, happier lifestyle.

That said, having a morning routine *is* important, however you choose to go about having one. When deciding on what kind of routine to go for, remember these rules:

- It has to work for *you* and your life
- Give yourself some time to try it out, but don't be afraid to drop it and try something better if it really isn't working for you
- Take responsibility—it's up to you and you alone to improve your life; nobody else can do it for you!

Why a Morning Routine is so Important

You might start implementing a morning routine for one reason and be pleasantly surprised that it has some positive side effects in other areas of your life. Discipline is funny like that—it has a tendency to spill over into other areas of your life. "Getting up on the right side of the bed" so to speak can prime the rest of your day for success. Mornings are important since they set the tone for everything that follows.

Before I set up a proper morning routine for myself, I wasted a lot of time, to put it mildly. I dragged myself out of bed (after snoozing my alarm clock more times than I care to admit) and then immediately went for coffee to cancel out the previous night's late bedtime. Then I'd procrastinate on all the things I knew I should be doing, run out of time, and be in a bad mood by the early afternoon. My productivity, my mood, and my overall wellbeing were always pretty low. A bad morning can start small, but it snowballs throughout the day.

With a solid morning routine, though, you put your best foot forward when you're at your brightest and freshest. You grab hold of the day with clear intention and focus, and *you steer it the way you want it to go* rather than passively reacting to whatever stress or obligations come your way. This means you're more focused, more aware, and getting more done. It's a different kind of snowball—you build your confidence and feeling of power in yourself, which inspires you to keep going, push through resistance, and feel proud of taking charge of your day. It's hard to imagine an area of life that isn't improved—relationships, physical health, finances, you name it.

How to Create a Morning Routine

Below I've listed five simple and practical changes you can make to your morning routine—starting from tomorrow. It's unwise to try to do too much at once. Instead, pick one or two at most and try it out for a few days. It takes time for a new habit to settle in. You need to try out a new habit for long enough that you can give it a fair shot, but also allow yourself to make any necessary tweaks and adjustments. What I'm saying is be patient—don't give up if it takes a few tries to get into a good momentum.

Tip 1: Have a Plan

If you *don't* have a plan and you wake up, what's the most likely thing you're going to end up doing?

Yup—it's probably a tossup between "stay in bed and mess around on my phone" or "fall asleep again." A lack of clarity can be a killer. If you have a loose plan (or no plan at all), what that means is that you're leaving the door wide open to excuses, dawdling, and procrastination. Don't rely on yourself to have the presence of mind and willpower to come up with a plan there and then as you wake up. It seems like a good idea to imagine yourself doing that *now*, but fast forward to tomorrow morning, when you're all cozy in bed and half asleep. Are you really going to be super excited to get out the to-do list and start planning your day?

Give yourself a break by making a plan and making it in advance. You need to know in crystal clear detail exactly what you're going to be doing from the moment your eyes open and the day starts. It's about being *intentional*. Neuroscientists and behavioral psychologists have discovered in study after study that writing down goals and vividly visualizing them, makes them far more likely to be achieved than plans and goals that are merely thought about.

Writing things down makes them more real for your brain and easier to encode and store. It's essentially a way of telling yourself, "This is really happening now." Sit down with a pen and paper and write down a timeline with your intended activities from the second you wake up. For example:

7:00 – Alarm goes off. Get up to go and turn it off. Immediately do some quick stretches and open the curtains and window. Take a deep breath of fresh air.

7:05 – Turn on the shower, and while it's warming up, quickly make the bed and straighten up the bedside table.

7:10 – Shower, shave, then get dressed (clothes laid out the night before).

7:30 – Make a cup of coffee and enjoy that while checking emails and making any last-minute adjustments to the schedule for the day.

8:00 – Make breakfast—overnight oats with a protein shake. Quickly unpack dishwasher and feed the cat.

9:00 – Start the day's work.

Now, you might read the above and think *that's a lot of detail*. And it is! But the truth is that once this little routine has been cemented as a habit, it can be carried out automatically with almost zero effort. Each step follows on from the last, none more taxing than having to brush your teeth. The point about being this deliberate and detailed is that you are setting a good foundation. After a week or so, you won't be checking your schedule to see what to do next—you'll just do it without thinking.

You may have noticed a few things in the above morning routine. Setting your alarm but then putting it far from the bed is a simple but very effective way of making sure that when it's time to get up, you get up! Don't even give yourself the option of hitting the snooze button. Put your phone in the next room so that when it buzzes, you get up. Then, you can set another alarm for five minutes' time, just to make sure you're not tempted to crawl back into bed.

A good trick is to put your alarm next to the following step in your routine. For example, you could put your phone near a window that you open to let light in (bright light will signal to your brain that it's time to get up and go) or in the kitchen where you begin your daily chores or make breakfast. You could put your phone in another room right next to your running shoes. This way, you wake up and your shoes are right there. You put them on, and you're right at the front door, ready for a quick fifteen-minute jog to wake you up. The idea is that all these events trigger one another like dominoes so you are carried along on your routine without much thought. In other words, it takes more effort not to follow your routine than to follow it. You may find yourself outside and on your run before you even have the chance to consider what excuses you're going to make for not doing it that morning.

Write down your morning schedule and take a look at each item, making sure that each one leads into and triggers the next.

Tip 2: Engage Your Body

When you wake up in the morning, the thing you're most conscious of is probably that your brain is still "booting up" and that you're a little groggy. But sleep is a complete physiological state, and it takes time for your entire system to wake up in the morning. You are not asleep one second and then awake the next. Your body moves through a complex and nuanced twenty-four-hour cycle of wakefulness. Waking up fully means coming to consciousness, but also ramping up your metabolism and getting your muscles and joints warmed up and active for the day after hours spent dormant.

In the example schedule we had above, you might have noticed that a few minutes of stretching was included pretty early on. You don't have to do a full, intense workout to get your blood pumping, though. In fact, the more gently you can wake up your system, the better. It's up to you how you want to include physical movement into your morning routine, but whatever you do, don't ignore your body in the morning. Waking up to immediately plonk yourself down in a work chair for eight hours is not exactly a recipe for good health! It's no surprise that people who do this don't have brilliant physical fitness, even if they faithfully do their afternoon workout.

Physical movement can start even before you get out of bed. When you wake, take a deep, deep breath and stretch out your arms and legs. Really take your time and relish it! Your body's circadian rhythm (sleep-wake cycle) is triggered and regulated by many different cues in the environment. One cue is exposure to natural sunlight, and another is movement.

It's not a good idea to rush into anything, though. If you plan to work out first thing in the morning, you'll need to build in a longer and more gradual warmup phase. Start with a gentle walk or jog before getting stuck into the main workout itself, or do some light yoga or Pilates. Be gentle with yourself—remember, just because you're mentally awake, it doesn't mean your body is ready to just spring into action without a warmup. Try one of the following:

- A few big stretches for your hips, shoulders, and back—do what comes naturally or choose a few you know work for you and your body
- A yoga routine—but avoid recorded things on screens, as this can be overly stimulating or distracting in the morning
- Take a walk outside
- Roll your ankle joints and your wrists and circle your neck around to loosen any tension

Each person has their own unique "chronotype," which is their personal circadian rhythm. In other words, some people are morning people and are their most focused and energized in the morning, preferring to go to sleep earlier. Others are groggy in the morning and tend to wake late, only hitting their peak later in the afternoon or even at night. They tend to stay up later and be more productive after lunch than before. People have different rhythms depending on the season, too, and women can vary in their energy levels depending on their monthly cycles.

It's worth recognizing your own preferences and limitations, working around them. You don't *have to* work out in the morning, but even if you're a night owl type, it's still worth doing some gentle stretching and walking. Does vigorous exercise before breakfast leave you feeling awful? Then just do it later!

A great idea is to combine a little physical activity in the morning with other healthy habits that get you off to the right start. Throw open the windows (the light will encourage melatonin production, which makes you feel more awake), fill your lungs with fresh air, or take a brisk walk while everything is still fresh and cool outside. You could also pair physical activity with a little mindfulness practice to get your head right before the day starts. Do your stretches along with a full "body scan" where you take the time to note how you feel, body and mind, and adjust accordingly. Note if you're feeling a little tired or under the weather, if your muscles are stiff, where your emotions are at, and so on. This will strengthen your self-awareness and make sure that you're able to consciously give yourself what you need each day.

Tip 3: Morning Workouts

Working out in the morning can be brilliant. There's nothing quite like knowing that you've already done an amazing, healthful workout . . . and it's only 9 a.m. The sense of accomplishment can be a real boost, energizing you for the rest of the day. It's not just psychological, though. Flooding your body with fresh, oxygenated blood, getting your joints and muscles moving, and getting your fill of feel-good endorphins all create a nice buzz in the morning. Exercise goes beyond physical health benefits. You'll also feel strong, capable, and proud as you challenge yourself and meet those challenges.

Getting your blood pumping and physically moving your body shift you into an active mindset (literally) where you're more likely to solve problems and move things forward. You can prove this to yourself any time you're slouching on a sofa somewhere— when you're horizontal and sluggish, do you really feel all that great about yourself? Or that confident about the future and your ability to steer it? Probably not.

As we said in the previous section, you don't necessarily need to work out in the morning if it really doesn't suit your physiology, your personality, or your lifestyle. But—what have you got to lose by trying it? Many people tell themselves that they're not "morning people" when the truth is that they've had such poor habits for so long, they mistakenly believe that they are naturally lazy and lethargic in the morning.

Now, before you even think of jumping in with the excuse that you hate the gym, think again. One of the biggest lies about getting more physically fit is that you need a lot of money or time to do it. The big sportswear companies and gyms want you to think this, sure, and perhaps unconsciously many of us accept this myth because it lets us off the hook: "I don't have the time!" "The nearest gym is miles away!" "I don't have any running shoes!"

Tell yourself right now: unless you are one hundred percent paralyzed from the top of your head to your toes, then you can be physically active. You don't need new gear, or a gym membership, or a DVD, or a personal trainer, or a whole new diet plan with supplements. Do you have a body? Then you can move it! In fact, the simpler you can keep things, the better. Switch your mind to solutions mode and don't listen to yourself when you come up with lazy excuses. ("It's my circadian rhythm that's to blame! I simply can't exercise in the mornings. Or in the evenings. Or . . . well, ever.")

- YouTube is a free resource splitting at the seams with exercise videos and educational content. Pick your favorite—there's barre ballet, Zumba-style dance classes, calisthenics, Pilates, yoga, boxing, and some retro Jane Fonda

27

aerobics videos from back in the day, if that's your thing
- Walk. It's the easiest, most effective way to get yourself moving. If you have an open field, try sprinting for some free, highly effective HIIT training
- If you don't have dumbbells, use milk or water jugs, bricks, cans, or other heavy things. Do tricep dips on a chair, pullups on a (sturdy) doorframe, or calf raises on the edge of your stairs. Be creative—your cavemen ancestors didn't need gym equipment!

It's not enough to sit on your butt all day, completely sedentary, and then do a brief thirty minute workout once before sitting down again. Workouts are great, but pay attention to your overall activity levels, too. You may be surprised to know that your "non-exercise activity thermogenesis" (i.e. NEAT, or all those calories you burn just by moving around in life) usually burns *more* calories per day than deliberate exercise workouts.

Read that again: the bulk of your fitness and energy expenditure is not in your thirty-minute or hour workout, but in all those smaller accumulating activities like housework, shopping, typing, standing, doing chores, or whatever.

So, try to get out of the idea that as long as you do your morning workout, you're good and can slob around for the rest of the day. Do your morning workout but don't forget to build in more activity elsewhere in your routine. Walk or cycle where you can, take the stairs, dig around in the garden, clean the house, play with your kids or the dog, make dinner, do some DIY or a hobby . . . you get the idea.

Tip 4: Getting Breakfast Right

You know the saying that "breakfast is the most important meal of the day"? Yeah, forget that. Unsurprisingly, this myth was orchestrated by breakfast cereal manufacturers decades ago, and the belief that we should all be eating breakfast has stuck ever since. We'll start this tip with a huge caveat: if you don't eat breakfast, never have eaten breakfast, and don't want to eat breakfast, then feel free to skip over this section. Just like with sleep, no two bodies are exactly the same, and some of us function better when we eat a little later in the day rather than first thing.

Intermittent fasting is now popular enough that many people are consciously choosing to avoid breakfast and start the day lighter and more clear-headed. And that's fine! So long as you are eating a balanced, healthy diet each day, skipping breakfast will do you no harm and indeed may have plenty of health benefits. Autophagy is the physiological state the body enters during fasting. Not only will fat start to be burned after around sixteen hours of fasting (lipolytic ketosis), but the body will also begin to "tidy up" damaged cells, regenerate the GI tract, and help you feel more mentally alert.

But if you *are* a person who eats breakfast, then you might like to take a closer look and see if you're doing the best you can with this daily habit. You would never start the day with an argument with your spouse, or deliberately seek out stressful news on your smartphone the second after waking up (okay, maybe you might), but eating a bad breakfast is just as harmful, if not more so.

Breakfast should be a hardworking meal for you. Is it carrying its weight, nutritionally speaking? Many experts recommend having a breakfast that is relatively high in protein and low in sugar or processed carbohydrates. So, no to sugary cereal, piles of fruit, or "healthy" granola bars that are really just candy in disguise. Yes to scrambled eggs, a protein smoothie, or natural peanut butter on wholewheat toast. Breakfast doesn't need to be big; plan to eat less than a third of your calories at this meal—for example, have a three-hundred calorie bowl of oats with some high-protein Greek yogurt if your daily intake is fifteen hundred calories.

Now that we've got the *what* covered, let's look at the *how*.

Unless you explicitly want to, try to avoid having to prepare complicated food in the morning, and instead have things set up so you can get breakfast sorted out quickly. Smoothies come together quickly if you keep your blender easily accessible and you have a ready store of frozen fruit in your freezer. You could make "overnight oats" that you prepare the night before and have ready and waiting in the morning (Google for about a billion different recipes and ideas), or you could even cook extra for dinner the night before and set aside some for leftovers.

When you eat, do your best not to rush. Don't eat and multitask—it's just a recipe for indigestion! Sit somewhere quiet and relish your meal without getting distracted by screens. Give yourself enough time in the morning to eat properly. It's another opportunity to be more mindful. You're not a robot, and you don't have to be your own drill sergeant to have a great morning routine. While we're on the subject of making time to actually enjoy your mornings, let's look at the final tip:

Tip 5: Cordon off Some Quiet Time

Some people start every morning in chaos. It's a mad, stressful dash; everyone's late, sleepy, or grumpy; and things are never quite done properly. Sound familiar?

If your mornings are currently . . . let's say, "challenging," then don't worry, it *is* possible to begin your days with calm tranquility instead. I promise. You absolutely need a plan (see tip 1), and you need to give yourself ample, realistic time frames to fulfil that plan. Being late causes anxiety, anxiety causes mistakes and more lateness, and round and round we go on the crazy morning carousel.

Though it might not seem like it from the long list of tasks we've mentioned in the tips above, your morning should ideally *not* be action packed and super intense. We've already seen that rushing into vigorous physical activity first thing in the morning is not going to feel great (and could cause injury) and that it's better to ease into your day gently and steadily. In the same way, your emotional state, your mood, and your overall cognitive clarity need time to wake up, too.

If you dive into emotionally stressful, overly stimulating, or unpleasant things immediately after you wake up, it goes without saying that you're laying the groundwork for a bad day. When making a big lifestyle change, it's tempting to go all out and hit your new commitments with as much vigor as you can muster. Wanting to smash our bad habits and chase our goals, we might start to see mornings as periods of *go go go*—you know, a little like a drill sergeant marching into your room and clanging a gong to wake you up at 4 a.m. to do a vigorous jog around the field. This might seem on the surface like a great way to get your mind into a disciplined, productive state . . . but it's really not.

Instead, see mornings as a time to set the tone and intention for the rest of the day. Start as you intend to continue. Don't be one of those people who loves complaining about how "busy" they are—if you are rushed and stressed every morning, that's simply a sign of poor planning and preparation. The more calm intention and focus you bring to your life, the less room there is for chaos, stress, and rushing.

We'll be looking at mindfulness and meditation in other sections of this book, but for now, think about how you could take a quiet moment to gather yourself and become aware. It doesn't have to be for all that long, either. Simply spend some quiet time alone, getting your body, heart, and mind calm and aligned for the day ahead.

- Listen to a feel-good podcast or beautiful music (avoid the news like the plague)
- Take a moment to journal a little, contemplate, or scribble down some thoughts and impressions
- Do a quiet, gentle hobby or take some time to put your living space in order
- Have a cup of coffee or tea outside and simply enjoy the sounds, sights, and smells

- Try a deep-breathing exercise
- Do a few stretches or a slow nature walk
- Take a moment to really savor your breakfast—don't do anything else, just enjoy it in the moment

If you find you're stressed about something scheduled for that day, now's the time to untangle and organize your thoughts. It'll be much easier for you to come up with creative solutions if you approach the issue with a calm, quiet mind. For emotionally difficult or draining times ahead, you can try visualization: close your eyes and vividly paint a picture in your mind's eye of how you will meet that challenge. See yourself facing any stressful or difficult moments with alert presence of mind. Play out what you want your responses to be that day before you are in the thick of it and are tempted to simply *react* to things happening around you. Affirmations and mantras can help, too. For example, "I am a capable and hard-working person, and today I trust myself to face any challenges without losing my composure."

Summary

- There is no optimal way to start your morning—the best morning routine is one that fits with *your* personal values, limitations, and goals.
- With a morning routine, you take charge of the day and steer it in the direction you want it to go. Start with one or two tweaks first, rather than changing everything all at once.
- Plan your morning the day before and draw up a detailed schedule.
- Even if you don't have a full workout, engage in some form of physical movement to wake up your body. Try stretching, deep breathing, walking, or yoga.
- If you do a morning workout, take your time to warm up properly. Morning workouts can set your day up for success.
- You don't have to eat breakfast—fasting in the morning can have incredible health and weight loss benefits. If you choose to have breakfast, though, plan it

the night before and go for something small, protein-packed, and convenient.

- Finally, don't rush in the mornings. A solid plan and enough time will ensure you move through your morning routine without chaos or stress. Deliberately factor in quiet time where you journal, plan the day ahead, contemplate, meditate, or simply enjoy breakfast or coffee outside while orienting to the day ahead.

Chapter 2: Dedication

What it Means to be Dedicated

When it comes down to it, dedication is about *commitment*.

It is when we purposefully and intentionally devote our time, energy, and attention to the things we most care about and value. When we have consciously made the decision for ourselves that we want to be better, or to make a change, it is a moment when we summon energy within ourselves to power that change.

Many of us can summon energy for a little while and make grand plans for the goals we'd like to achieve. But the trick is also to *sustain* that energy over time, long after the initial enthusiasm for the goal has fizzled off and the hard work begins. Dedication is the promise you make to yourself that you will continue despite difficulties and obstacles. This promise keeps you going from the moment you begin, through the difficult slog, and out the other side, when you achieve your goal. It's a commitment.

Why Dedication Matters

When it comes to leading a healthier lifestyle, being dedicated is actually non-negotiable. You simply cannot make and maintain any real lifestyle change if you don't have the dedication required. I'd like to say that there are tips and tricks to make the process easier (in fact, you're holding a book of tips and tricks in your hands right now), but the truth is, none of it matters unless you make that decision to actually do them, not just once, but over and over again.

Being dedicated doesn't just help you achieve your goals, uproot bad behaviors, and replace them with better ones. It boosts your confidence, too. When you hold firm in your principles and stick to your word, you feel strengthened and proud about your ability to follow through. You feel more capable and empowered—what else could you achieve if you put your mind to it? Feeling this way, you have the self-respect and pride needed to set goals and standards for yourself, knowing you have what it takes to get there. This is a priceless feeling, and in a way, it's much more valuable than simply losing a few pounds!

How to be More Dedicated

Being dedicated is about what you **do**. It's about action. But it starts inside you, with a rock-solid commitment. You need your inner commitment *and* your conscious action to work together. Action without any thought or planning is meaningless, and good intentions that are never realized through action are useless.

Learning to bring more dedication into your life means processing each of your thoughts, hopes, plans, and dreams through one criterion: it has to be actionable. Whether you are trying to eat better and get more fit, whether you want more discipline at work, or whether you're trying to live a healthier, more balanced life in general, sooner or later you will need to make your intention a reality and act.

In the last chapter, we spoke about starting the day on the right foot by designing the perfect morning routine. But when you are dedicated, you need to continually renew your commitment to being better all throughout the day. Your day will be a string of decisions, i.e. a constant conveyor belt of choices giving you the opportunity to move toward your goal or further away from it. Your dedication will help you make the best of those choices.

How can you be more dedicated? Keep translating your thoughts into action.

Tip 6: Tiny Changes Add Up

I know you want to overhaul your life completely. I know how tempting it is to make a big, flashy change and do a drastic life makeover that solves all your problems once and for all. But resist this tendency—

it's a trap! The less glamorous truth is that change, real change, happens in tiny increments. There is no overnight transformation, but rather a long, long stream of steady improvements, some so small you won't even be sure you're making progress at all some days.

What keeps you going? Dedication!

Take a look at your daily routine. Ask yourself, "What's the smallest sustainable change I can make right now?" Note that it's not the biggest, most impressive, or most exciting change. It's the *smallest sustainable* one. It's the one you can easily do for the next days, weeks, months, forever.

For example, you could switch out your full fat milk for skim milk in your morning coffee. A tiny, almost imperceptible change. But over the course of a year, or a lifetime, you save an impressive number of calories and hence spare yourself that weight gain. That's the trick: the most impressive results often come about with the changes that seem kind of unremarkable in the moment.

The secret is that you *persist* with these small changes, and they add up.

- Get a standing desk so you're more active during the workday and being less sedentary
- Make substitutions to your diet rather than eliminations: wholewheat pasta instead of plain, fresh fruit instead of candy, water instead of sweetened drinks, salad instead of fries
- Remember NEAT (non-exercise activity thermogenesis)? Keep moving. Instead of taking the car for a quick drive, walk or cycle instead. Do your own housework. Place dumbbells around the house for a quick set here and there during gaps in other tasks
- Put a water bottle on your desk so you're always reminded to drink throughout the day

Now, it would be a mistake to jump in and try one of the above without really thinking about it. Remember that the goal is to bring our commitments and intentions to life with action. Just taking any old action because it seems like a good idea is likely to fizzle out. You need to build into your life those actions that genuinely align with your values and the goals you have for yourself. This means that it's impossible to say what *you personally* should be doing in your life right now. Only you know that!

But here's a quick way to determine what small actions you can commit to taking each day to build healthful habits:

1. First, identify your desired end point or goal. Let's imagine it's to join a friend on a massive mountain hike in a few months' time.
2. Now, translate that goal into three concrete action steps that you can do *every day*. You might decide that you will take a daily walk after dinner each evening, you'll stop having desserts or seconds after dinner each evening, and you'll do five minutes of stretching before bed.

Simple, right? Will these actions alone suddenly make it possible to complete the big hike? No. But they pave the way. In two weeks' time, once you've consistently sustained these tasks, you can dial it up: go for longer walks (or make them jogs), tidy up your diet further and do longer exercise sessions. It's okay to start small if it means you keep going—if you had started out by jumping into a two-hour exercise session on Monday morning, you would have only burnt yourself out and given up by Wednesday.

Tip 7: Identify Your Weak Spots—Then Fortify Them

You need to build a new, healthier life on top of the life you already have. And to do that, it works best to identify the places that could most use some attention right now and target them first. What could you be doing better?

With enough presence of mind, you might start to look at your daily routine and see opportunities for improvement. Become curious about how small tweaks can make big changes. For example, many people have successfully cut down their sugar and junk food consumption by realizing that "if it's in the house, I'll eat it . . . so I just won't have it in the house!" They became mindful of their behavior and stepped in to change it.

But the first step is to be mindful. Maybe you notice you always spend Saturdays at the mall. Could you walk instead of drive to the mall? If not, could you park far away in the parking lot so you have to walk closer? Could you spend more time standing and walking in the mall? You may be struggling to find ways to squeeze in a daily walk in the park when really, you already have the opportunity to do more walking right there—you just need to notice it and capitalize on it.

You already know so many of the healthy habit tips out there—do your shopping on a full stomach so you're not tempted to buy junk food, use a basket and not a trolley, deliberately stick to the outer edges of the shop where the fresh produce is, and so on . . . But these are all generic. They may apply to you, and they may not. It's far better to look at your unique and individual life and see what needs to be addressed. You may find that your efforts are better rewarded when they are tailored to your life as it stands right now. For example:

- You notice that you never, ever stick to a gym schedule and usually let your membership lapse. So, you drop the idea of going to the gym and instead sign up for dance classes three times a week, and other times just work out at home . . . which you love more and end up actually doing
- You notice that you usually end up making bad food decisions when you've had a few drinks. So, you dedicate yourself to having non-alcoholic drinks only
- You notice that you procrastinate most when you're tired and it's late in the afternoon. So, you schedule all your work (or most of it) for the

mornings, knowing that you're more likely to get it done then

Dedication comes from knowing what your goals are and committing to taking the actions necessary to bridge the gap between where you are and where you want to be. Zoom in on a problem in your own daily life (for example, always being late in the morning or overeating) and get curious about it.

What is your ultimate goal?
What concrete actions can you take right now to reach that goal slowly?
And finally, what is standing in the way of you taking those actions?

You can fortify your weak spots by making it as easy as possible to do the right thing. Remove everything that makes it hard for you to follow through on your commitment. If you notice time and time again that you can't trust yourself to prepare healthy meals, then arrange for a food delivery service. If you notice that you always eat too much at family gatherings, limit your time there, bring your own food, or make sure you're sufficiently distracted with other things that you're not constantly tempted.

Tip 8: Making Work Work for You

In reading the previous section, maybe you thought, "That's great and all, but I don't always have control over these things, like at work." Maybe you're desperately trying to clean up your diet but work in an office where birthday cake is passed around twice a week with heavy pressure to eat some. Maybe your commute takes up big blocks of your time that you could be exercising or relaxing, or maybe you can't turn down the endless after-work drinks that are starting to cost you sleep—not to mention money!

Then what?

Rest assured, it's always possible to make healthy changes to your lifestyle and take charge of your wellbeing no matter what your work situation is. But again, it takes awareness, dedication, and the commitment to being consistent day after day.

- Pack a lunch instead of buying one. It's healthier, cheaper, and will save you time, plus it gives you complete control over what you eat. Prepare it the night before. You can batch-prepare them or simply make extra food for dinner and pack the leftovers

- Get up and move during your lunch break—don't sit at your desk. Take a walk, even if it's just to get some fresh air outside or stroll around the building

- Avoid caffeine after lunch, or switch to decaf either completely or partially. Caffeine can be great for work performance, but it's not for everyone and can exacerbate anxiety

- Prepare a healthy snack stash so you're not tempted to nibble on unhealthy things. Include fruit, nuts, or protein bars—but check their calorie count first!

- Have an hourly routine—for every hour of work, get up to stretch your legs, drink some water, rest your eyes, mindfully check in with yourself, or do some desk stretches

- Have boundaries. It may be hard at first to turn down invitations or offers, but firmly and politely say no and keep saying no. If you assert a boundary and really mean it, people will eventually respect that—you may even inspire them to make healthier changes too!

- Boundaries extend to time and resources, too. Be firm about not taking work home with you or checking messages after work hours. Same thing goes with expensive fundraisers and the like. While this may feel incredibly difficult, a huge part of your health is your mental wellbeing—consider an act of self-care to put your needs as a priority!

- In extreme cases, you might need to seriously reconsider your job or work environment if you consistently feel that it undermines your health and wellbeing. See what can be done to restructure your workday, or look for another position

- If there's an entrenched unhealthy culture at work, see if you can inspire change—suggest a group healthy eating challenge, a fun run, or argue for better snacks in the cafeteria

Summary

- Dedication is about making a promise to yourself to systematically rework old habits and thought patterns and replace them with better, healthier ones. Dedication means committing to following through with your goals, regardless of the obstacles in the way.

- Dedication matters because change is uncomfortable, and it takes energy and focus to shift us out of our status quo. Dedication helps us feel confident in our ability to do better, and fortifies our willpower.

- Being more dedicated is about taking your goals and bringing them to life by *taking concrete action*. Break goals down into small steps and act toward them every day.

- Remember that baby steps are more effective than quantum leaps. Make the smallest sustainable change possible, not the biggest change, since this is what adds up to big rewards in the long run.

- To start making progress and gaining momentum, begin with the "lowest hanging fruit." Identify your weak spots first and take action to replace those bad habits. This will give you the highest return on your efforts and motivate you to keep going.

- It can be especially tough to develop healthy habits in the workplace, so make sure you have a plan in place for how to keep your dedication going at work. If something's not working, ask, "How can I *make* this work?"

Chapter 3: Focus and Mentality

What to Focus On

You're probably noticing a pattern here—real change takes awareness, dedication, and consistency. Becoming healthier is not a single event that happens once and never again. Rather, it's something we constantly work on. We stay dedicated even when there are temptations all around. We stay dedicated even when others try to undermine us. We stay dedicated even when faced with our own blind spots, weaknesses, and bad habits. Starting with a structured, healthy morning routine, and moving through the day with commitment and regular check-ins, we arrive at an essential part of the change process: our mindset.

Whether you call it your attitude, your approach, your perception, or your mindset, the things that you choose to focus on will invariably be the things that end up dominating your life. It really is as simple as that: focus on negativity, lack, and what you dislike, and you amplify these things in your life. Focus on the positive and what you can do to grow and learn, and that's what your life becomes filled with.

Life changes when we take action to change it.
Taking action comes from the goals we set.
We form our goals because of what we focus on.
Our focus is determined by our attitude or mindset.

So, the root of change, then, is mindset.

Why Mindset Matters

Our attitude is a narrative frame of reference that organizes how we think and feel, how we make sense of life, how we interpret events, and what we think is possible. It affects everything, including how we communicate, how we appraise risk, our response to adversity . . . and how we set goals. It goes a lot deeper than simply "be positive," although, to be honest, being positive is a pretty good start!

Staying Optimistic and Having a Positive Mindset

Being positive doesn't mean you ignore or downplay problems—it just means you keep your eyes and ears open for solutions to those problems, knowing that there is always something you can do to improve the situation. Your focus is on solutions, not problems.

Being positive doesn't mean you are unrealistic, either. It means you shift your focus from what can't be done and what isn't working, to what *can* be done and what *is* working. If we fail or stumble, we ask how we can be better next time, rather than dwelling on the fact that we didn't make it this time. It's a matter, again, of **focus**. What

57

you focus on becomes bigger. So what do you want to focus on?

Work on your mindset and everything else follows. But if you have a negative mindset, it won't matter much that you do all the right things. The following are some tips for keeping a positive, empowered mindset as you make changes to your life.

Tip 9: Have Daily, Weekly, and Monthly Milestones

Don't try to change everything at once. Instead, take all your energy and willpower and focus it into one or two big changes at a time so you can narrow down your attention on them and get things done more effectively (and more easily). There are tons of things you do every day right now without having to think about them. In time, you can make it so that you also do healthy, good habits everyday in exactly the same way: automatically and without much effort.

Its not enough to make a goal that will be achieved "someday," or set yourself a five-year plan and then put your feet up. Your goals need to include short-, medium-, and long-term objectives, and you need to regularly give yourself the chance to reappraise them and adjust as you go.

The more milestones, the better. Let's say you're trying to eat more fruit and veggies every day. Narrow your focus by deciding what this actually means—how many servings? How many grams or ounces of fruit and veggies? What kind of fruit and veggies, and when, and how will you eat them? Make specific and concrete goals. For example, you commit to eating some kind of fruit or veggies at every meal of the day for a week. Then, the week after, you give yourself the goal of five servings of a certain size. At the end of the month, your goal is to have an unbroken streak of days where you've consistently met your smaller goal.

Let's tie this back to a positive mindset: the more you experience the sensation of achieving a goal, even a small one, the more encouraged and positive you'll feel about yourself. You'll be telling your unconscious mind that not only is this really possible, but that you're busy doing it right now. When you reach a milestone, pause to give yourself a pat on the back, acknowledging your hard work so that you cement it in your mind with praise and validation.

Don't make the mistake of assuming that small goals don't mean much—they do! Think of it this way, if you have to wait and wait for months or years before you can celebrate your progress, aren't you going to get bored and unmotivated? Isn't your enthusiasm going to wane with time as you realize you keep working hard but for no reward? The trick, then, is to give yourself rewards. It's much easier to carry on your path with purpose and energy if you are regularly stopping to appreciate your progress and celebrate a little. This isn't permission to stop, of course, but it's encouragement to keep going.

- Count your fitness goals in small increments, like the number of pushups, sit-ups, or steps done in one day. If you don't do well on one day, that's okay. You can still see an overall trend in the weekly or monthly average. Keep a visual track on these goals, like logging daily steps on a chart, to monitor your progress and feel proud of your achievement. Seeing this log visually everyday will keep you motivated

- Plan a time at the end of each week or month (Sundays work) where you see how well you did and decide whether to set a new goal or adjust the current one

- Tell others what your plans are so you feel supported and encouraged. They will also help you stay accountable to yourself and be there to celebrate with you when you achieve your goals

Tip 10: Healthy vs Unhealthy Rewards

So, praising yourself when you reach your milestones is great, but be careful—"rewards" can be a slippery slope. If you train yourself to know that doing well earns you a reward, then naturally, you're incentivized to do just so. What you don't want, however, is to become dependent on that reward or worse, for that reward to be precisely the kind of bad habit or behavior that undoes all your hard work.

The rationale behind a reward is to make the healthy behavior or habit seem more appealing, to increase its value in your eyes, and to make it more of an obvious choice. Sure, you could just *force* yourself to do right by sheer power of the will, but this takes a lot of effort, isn't sustainable . . . and just all around sucks for the person doing it! Rewards teach your brain that doing the healthy thing actually feels good, and that you *want* to do the healthy thing. You do this by making an association with the desired behavior and good feelings to make that behavior more attractive and repeatable in the future. (I bet you can see now the wisdom of having small, more frequent opportunities for reward built in to celebrate every day—more opportunities to cement your desired behavior!).

- Don't underestimate the value of simply praising yourself. Tell someone what you're proud of accomplishing. Print yourself out a certificate to mark the pounds lost or miles jogged, and hang it on the wall! Tell yourself, out loud and to the mirror, "You did a good job." Don't focus on your fixed characteristics, but on the effort and determination you put in—because those are the things that count and the things you want to encourage. This is where the possibility of change lies.

- Accumulate evidence of your achievements. Keep a whiteboard where you put a tick for every day you follow through on your healthy habit, or for every pound lost, or for every step closer to your goal, however you conceive it. Keep that visual reminder where you can see it—especially when you're feeling tempted to forget your commitment!

- Once you've achieved a goal, consider buying yourself a little present. Just make sure this isn't an unhealthy snack, of course. If you're trying to eat better, think of treats like a luxurious kind of tea, a beautiful box of fresh berries, a new book, tickets to do something fun with people you love, a little potted plant . . . you get the picture.

- Rewards don't have to be material. If you've worked hard, it's fine to take some time off and relax. If you can, take the day off, go out somewhere new, catch up on socializing with friends, or give yourself permission to indulge in a hobby.

This is a chapter about mindset. The mindset you have when it comes to rewards and meeting goals matters a lot. Too many people fail in their diet and exercise plans because they think, consciously or unconsciously, that what they are doing is only temporary, or that it's a bit like a punishment. As soon as they achieve their goal, they intend to go right back to what they were doing before—i.e. the "reward" of achieving their goals is to go right back to square one and pretend they haven't evolved! Can you see how illogical this is?

If you see your efforts to improve yourself as a boring, painful slog, you won't be able to keep it up for long. If your heart's not in it, if you're doing it out of a sense of obligation (or don't even know why you're doing it), you're setting yourself up to fail. Remember that what you focus on becomes bigger—if you keep focusing on how annoying and difficult and scary change is, what do you think will happen? You'll convince yourself it's not worth it and stop. But if you frame your actions as a gift you're giving yourself, as a sign of self-respect, and as an exciting but challenging new adventure you're going on, that changes things completely.

It's worth keeping an eye on your mindset. Keep telling yourself, "I want to change. I'm not doing this for anyone but myself. I know it will be challenging, but I can do it. It will get easier . . ." and so on. Don't complain or grumble. Don't act like others are forcing you to make changes. And when you have a reward, have it not because it's bribery to behave better, but because you are celebrating the awesome new person you're becoming.

Tip 11: Thinking about Food

Let's be honest, you could fill this entire book talking about "healthy eating" and how to do it. Or you could read any of the seemingly billions of diet and nutrition books out there. Low carb, keto, vegan, intermittent fasting, Mediterranean, GI diet . . . there's no way of eating that someone hasn't claimed is the One True Way. But that means there's a frustrating amount of conflicting and confusing advice out there for those of us who simply want to be healthier.

Don't worry, I'm not about to tell you which diet is the ultimate perfect diet and shun all the others. The truth? They all work to some degree.

What do all the different types of diet have in common? Think about it. They all recommend eating different foods at different times of day in different combinations for different reasons. Even though they're all quite different from each other, people can and do find great results. So, a high-carb vegan can lose weight and feel amazing eating a diet that is the exact opposite of a carnivorous, low carb keto fanatic who eats once every twenty-four hours—and also feels amazing.

What do they have in common? Mindset. Not the same mindset, no, but they all share a commitment and a focus to following certain principles, and the dedication needed to do that. They all rely on a degree of *mindfulness* about what is eaten and why, and a certain amount of conscious *control* over that. You can see where this is going: your success with eating isn't about the kind of diet you follow per se, but about the discipline, dedication, and conscious intention that you bring to following it.

That said, it's up to you to look honestly at where you are now, clarify where it is you want to go, choose a plan of action that suits your needs and limitations, and then commit to yourself that you will do what it takes to get there. The following are some ideas:

- Have a goal for each day's food intake. For a while, I found it helpful to focus on fruits and veggies. I kept a running tally of how many I was eating and tried to eat at least five servings a day from at least three color groups. Your goal could be to include a quality source of protein with each meal, or to consistently avoid refined carbohydrates.

- Counting calories is sometimes criticized, but it's still an easy and proven effective way to track your intake. Try what works for you—install a phone or desktop app where you can log your food, or keep a written record. Have a food budget where you know not to go over a certain limit per meal. Or you could have a rule such as "never eat more than six hundred calories per meal, or go over one thousand calories by lunchtime"

- Piece together your own eating manifesto—a bit like a personal set of commandments tailored for you. It's your choice what you focus on. You may be more concerned about non-processed food, want to eat more nutritious things, or cut the volume of food you eat in general. Write this manifesto out and keep it somewhere visible—like on the fridge.

- As before, identify your weak spots and take action *before* you're faced with temptation. Google restaurants beforehand to find places that will serve you food you're happy with, or bring your own healthy food to a potluck—or offer to cook for everyone!

- Don't beat yourself up if you slip now and again. Don't turn a little mistake into a big one by thinking, "Well, I've messed up now. I might as well throw everything out the window." Expect that you *will* slip up sometimes. Forgive yourself quickly and just carry on. As soon as you can, take a concrete step in the right direction again—you'll feel much better than if you wallow in self-criticism.

Tip 12: Automate

When you are focused, you need to tune out a lot of unnecessary noise and stimuli and zoom in on just the thing you're most interested in. That's why discipline often comes with being able to resist temptation and distraction—to tune out irrelevant data and focus only on what's really important.

At the start of your quest to live a healthier lifestyle, it can feel like the day is filled with wall-to-wall choices. You may feel like you have to reinvent the wheel with everything—the choice of what to eat, what not to eat, what activity to do, when to do it can seriously drain your mental resources. But willpower is a finite quantity. If you blow it all on deciding what kind of breakfast cereal to buy at the store, you may feel so drained and decision fatigued that you later make a regrettable choice out of tiredness or impatience.

One way to preserve your willpower resources and avoid "analysis paralysis" is to automate. This means taking as many of your choices as possible out of your hands. You want to build a life where you *automatically do the right thing* without having to think too much or spend too much effort. This frees you up to fight the big discipline monsters elsewhere.

So, how do you automate? Let's look at an example of someone trying to drink more water in their daily lives. It's a hassle to saddle yourself with the constant thought of "I should drink more water" all throughout the day. It just takes up too much mental bandwidth. Instead, set a repeating reminder on your phone, once, that tells you to drink a big glass of water. Then, forget about it! You spend a tiny amount of effort one time (setting the alarm) versus relying on your memory and discipline again and again every day.

You could also decide to put water bottles in literally every room of your home, and in your car. Wherever you are, it's easy to drink. You can always *see* a water bottle, so you don't need to remember anything. So, you idly take a sip. A little upfront effort means that you stick to your commitment and develop habits—all without having to use force or excessive discipline and willpower.

The above can be done with other things you want to make sure you take, eat or drink daily. Put vitamins next to your bed in plain view so you know to take them when you go to sleep or wake up. Or consider putting them next to your toothbrush—you don't forget to brush your teeth, right? If you're trying to eat more fruit and veggies in your life, have a mini fruit bowl on your desk at work. If you feel like a snack, it's far easier to just grab a nice apple or banana than get up, walk somewhere else, and potentially spend money to buy a less healthy snack. What you've done is made the desirable habit easier to perform than the undesirable habit. Now, this won't mean that you'll magically start wanting fruit and only fruit, but it will go a long way to cementing that behavior in your daily routine and making it more likely.

Habits tends to form over the course of three weeks or more. Until a behavior is cemented as habit, it will take effort, concentration, and discipline to perform. Once the behavior is embedded as a habit, though, it takes far less effort—or none at all. By using automation, you are making sure you keep doing the behavior during that crucial window period when it's not yet a habit. Ask yourself, *how can I make the desired behavior as easy as possible?*

- You could **delegate**. For example, give your cigarettes or unhealthy snacks to someone else and tell them to hide them from you when trying to quit. The decision is out of your hands
- Put up a **non-negotiable barrier**. Go to a cash bar but without any cash if you're trying to stop yourself from

drinking. Install an app on your laptop and phone that prevents you from browsing the internet after a certain hour, to stop yourself wasting time online late at night and getting insomnia. Put a lock with a timer on your kitchen cupboards to stop yourself from rummaging around for a midnight snack

- **Connect the desired behavior to an already established habit**. You always brush your teeth in the morning, so put your vitamins next to your toothbrush so you can take them right after you brush your teeth. You use the momentum of one habit to power a new one

There are no shortcuts, no, but automating gets the job done without you breaking too much of a sweat. It's about taking raw willpower out of the equation and letting your environment make some good choices for you on your behalf.

Tip 13: Have a Manifesto

In the same spirit of trying not to reinvent the wheel, let's consider another way to save time and effort: have a personal set of rules. When you're trying to learn a new behavior and change your lifestyle, you are faced with choices. Cake or no cake? Gym or TV? Now, you could sit there each time and weigh up the pros and cons and make an informed decision. But this takes time and, as we've seen, will quickly deplete your energy.

One way to automate your decision-making process is to have a set of rock-solid rules and principles. This is like making a decision once and then simply applying that every time you are faced with a new problem or situation. This simplifies things and takes away the need to analyze every fresh decision—not to mention give you less opportunity to dream up excuses!

How should you behave? Simply follows the rules you've set for yourself. For a very simple example, you can set the rule, "I don't do work for free." If a new client comes along and asks for free work, you simply say no and move on. No deliberation, no ifs and buts, just no and move on.

Having such a manifesto is like having a behavioral operating manual for yourself that makes decisions for you. In the heat of the moment, you can convince yourself to go the wrong way, you can make up excuses, you can forget your commitment, and so on. But your manifesto, your list of rules, stays the same. It can be a relief to know that as long as you follow your own rules, you're on the right path. Don't stress the big picture—just put your head down and focus on the task in front of you.

A manifesto is also just the thing to help you set boundaries:

- I don't have second helpings of dinner
- I don't answer work calls on the weekend
- I don't say yes to a request if it means I have to undermine my own needs
- I don't drink anything that's not water or tea

76

- I don't maintain friendships with people who lie to me
- I don't eat processed food

The above helps you conserve your resources, assert your boundaries, and be crystal clear about who you are and what you're committed to. People and situations *will* press on these boundaries (and let's face it, so will you), but they are always there, providing clarity and guidance. Take the time now to draw up your own personal "ten commandments" when it comes to lifestyle. Think about the things you want to say yes to and the things you always want to refuse (but may find difficult in the moment). Think about your values, principles, and the commitment you've made to yourself.

Having a strong sense of focus and a healthy mindset mean being able to clearly identify what you care most about, and having the courage to ignore or downplay the rest. Don't beat yourself up if you don't always manage to follow your own rules; these things take practice. Don't be afraid ether of making updates as you go. But give yourself the chance to go out into the world with intact boundaries and principles and see what happens. Learning to say no, to put your foot down, or to forcefully turn your attention away from one thing and onto another takes time—but like any habit, it does get easier.

Summary:

- When making improvements to your life, your focused and positive mindset is one of your greatest assets. Rather than being blindly "positive," you can simply become aware of where your focus and attention are going, and what you're choosing to create for yourself. Focus on solutions, not problems. Make it work.

- Regular milestones are necessary to keep up your motivation and focus. Schedule mini-milestones or rewards daily, weekly, and monthly. Take the time to acknowledge progress.

- When rewarding yourself, do so in a way that doesn't undermine your progress. Remember that you're celebrating your

78

better self, and rewards should help you enjoy your healthier life, not pull you back to your old, unhealthy life.

- *All* diet philosophies have some value— what makes them work is your positive mindset, your dedication, and your consistent action. Whatever diet you choose, it will succeed if you practice some form of control, and if you're mindful of your consumption.

- Willpower and energy are finite. To preserve them, automate certain choices so it's easy to automatically make the right choice and harder to make the wrong one.

- Piece together a personal healthy living manifesto of rules that help you decide how to act. This helps you set boundaries, banish excuses, and turn down temptation.

Chapter 4: Night Routine

For all the good reasons you want a morning routine, you want a nighttime routine. In the morning, you gear up, set your intention for the day, and fine tune your laser focus so that day is everything it can be. At night, though, the process switches to concluding what has already happened during the day so you can set things to rest, have a good night's sleep, and start fresh again the next day.

Something to consider: if you don't think you're a "morning person" the real problem might be that you are in fact having bad evenings that then reflect in difficult mornings. It's not impossible to have a brilliantly productive and calm morning when you've had a bad time the night before, but it's incredibly difficult. Think of your evenings as setting the stage for the day that follows.

What Kind of Routine Should I have at Night?

Any routine that lets you cement the good and learn from the bad from the day just passed is a good night routine. Similarly, just as a morning routine helps you wake up and start your engines, a night routine helps you wind them down again and ease into deep rest for the night. You should have a routine that is tailor-made to you and your goals and is realistically possible for you. It should be like a perfect full stop at the end of a great, productive day.

What You do Before Bed Matters—Here's Why

If you start your day in a stressful rush, you carry that energy with you into everything else you do, adopting a mindset that's exactly what you don't want when trying to live a healthy, purpose-driven life. If you have chaotic or stressful nights, insomnia, or simply pass out from exhaustion without taking the time to digest the day, you're putting yourself in that same mindset . . . and that will carry over into the next morning.

It's very easy to set up a continual loop, with bad mornings leading to bad evenings leading to bad mornings again. Paying conscious attention to exactly how you spend your evenings, however, gives you a degree of control over your thoughts, feelings, and actions at this time of day.

It's too difficult to try to make sweeping changes to your life when it's late at night and you're tired and tapped out. You need to plan ahead and have a habitual routine cycle that you flow through, one that optimizes your days rather than wastes them.

How to Get Started with a Good Night Routine

The process is not that different from setting up a morning routine. Make small changes at first and think carefully about not just your mind and emotions, but your body and where it is in its natural sleep/wake cycle. Build in enough quiet contemplative time so you can gather yourself with mindful attention. Then, you can direct your attention as you please, rather than getting carried away reacting to every new stimulus that comes your way. As before, a good place to start is with all the things you know you're already doing incorrectly. Go to bed too late? Your first challenge is to start inching that bedtime back. Scroll on devices in bed? Your focus is to create a zone of device-free calm before sleeping.

Tip 14: Make the Most Impactful Changes First

This is a tip that really applies to anything in life—begin with those actions and interventions that are most impactful and will bring you the highest return, i.e. go for the low-hanging fruit first. Look and see if you can identify the single worst habit you have in the evenings. What is the one thing you're doing that's causing the most trouble? Examples:

- You say you want to sleep at 10 p.m. but push it and push it and push it until it's 1 a.m. and you're bleary eyed and exhausted but still sitting in front of the TV. You wake up exhausted
- You "doomscroll" on your smartphone while in bed till your eyes burn and you're completely stressed, then have restless nights or even nightmares
- Out of boredom, you indulge in some late-night ice cream that interferes with your digestion and ruins your carefully planned diet for the whole day

Where is your biggest room for improvement in the evenings? Only you can say. But my guess is that you, like most people, probably go to bed far later than you should, or than is healthy. If you're consistently getting fewer than eight hours of sleep per night, or your sleep habits are all over the place, a great first step is to nail down a consistent bedtime that you stick to no matter what.

Going to sleep at the same time every night is, for most of us, the single most effective change we can make to our routines. Some people view going to bed almost like a battle; they procrastinate, perhaps because deep down, they're unsatisfied with how the day went and want to exert that tiny little bit of control by staying up when they shouldn't. Perhaps they don't want to face the next day. Whatever the reasons, you need to understand that deliberately depriving yourself of healthy, regular sleep is one of the quickest ways to self-sabotage and undermine all your grand plans for the following day.

It takes a little discipline at first. Set a time you're happy with and get into bed by that time, no excuses. Probably, if you're a chronic under sleeper, you won't fall asleep instantly. That's fine. Tell yourself you don't *have to* fall asleep, but you can't do anything else, like scroll on your phone or watch TV. Just stay peacefully in bed. This won't work, of course, unless you're also diligently getting up at the same time each morning. Don't let your wake-up time creep later and later to accommodate late bedtimes. Wake up when you say you will. You'll be tired during the day—but then you'll sleep on time the next night, and the vicious cycle will start to crack.

Good sleep hygiene is about knowing that you need to protect and maintain good habits around sleep, just as surely as you would around diet and exercise. Good sleep hygiene includes:

- Sleeping in a sufficiently dark room—get blackout curtains if it's too light. If that's not possible, try a sleep mask
- Your room should also be cool and comfortable—keep the windows slightly ajar for some fresh air flow
- Make sure your mattress is in good shape and properly supporting you,

as is your pillow. This is one area of life well worth investing in!

- Go for natural fibers for bedding and sleep clothes. Make sure they're clean, soft, and not too hot, cold, or restrictive
- If noise is a problem, use earplugs
- Don't drink too much liquid the few hours before bed to avoid nighttime bathroom breaks
- Avoid anything overly stimulating before bed, including caffeine (obviously!), but also any media or reading that stresses you out, arguments with other people, vigorous exercise, bright lights, or loud noises. Start winding down around thirty minutes to an hour before your chosen sleep time

The thing is, your body already has a built-in biological clock. Good sleep hygiene is simply there to support it. Making changes may feel hard at first, but once you slip into a healthy, comfortable rhythm, it will be easy and automatic. You may not even realize just how accustomed you had gotten to feeling groggy and irritable when you first start having good sleep every night. All those things you want—mental clarity, calmness, and positive mindset—will be much easier if you're rested and recovering well every night. And it all starts with simply committing to going to bed the same time each night!

Tip 15: Make Time for Reflection

The evenings are times of great opportunity. But most of us are too exhausted and fed up to make much of these opportunities. Sometimes we've had a long day and we just want to veg out with some junk food and not think about anything. But by doing so, we miss out on the chance to check in with ourselves, to appraise our progress, and to generally reflect on everything that's happened that day.

This is no idle contemplation—when we pause to reflect, we are *mentally digesting*. We process what has occurred, make minor course corrections, and ask mindfully what

89

we need to do next time round. We take a moment to feel proud of what we've accomplished, but we also analyze and file away anything that could have been better. This essentially sieves through the day and finds the gold nuggets so you can make informed decisions about what you want to do the next day.

You can do this by simply sitting quietly with yourself, but writing things down has the advantage of helping you be more organized and deliberate. What you focus on will change day to day, but here are some questions to get the reflection process going:

- Did you complete everything on your to-do list? If not, can you see *why*? Think of concrete steps to take to ensure that that same obstacle doesn't sabotage you tomorrow
- How was your state of mind throughout the day? Were you reactive and chaotic, calm and composed, bored, irritable, content? What stands out? What can you learn

from especially pleasurable or difficult moments? We can't always analyze these things in the moment, but at night, we have the chance to slowly unpack events and look at them closely

- Can you identify five things that you're grateful for today, no matter how small? Fostering gratitude keeps you in a positive, open frame of mind that's geared toward more creative problem solving, more self-compassion, and better communication
- What did you do well today? Zoom in on exactly why you were able to do so and ask how you can keep that going. Congratulate yourself—be glad whenever you rise to the challenge of being a better person!
- Note down some things you are looking forward to tomorrow, and think of how you will optimize on that—do you need to prepare or simply to make sure you're being appreciative and focused on it?

- Think of the things coming up tomorrow that will be challenging and do the same. What can you do to prepare yourself and make sure you're responding according to your values and goals? Use visualization to "rehearse" your attitude to this upcoming challenge, or try some affirmations

- If something is weighing heavily on your mind, it might not be possible to resolve everything that evening. Don't allow it to disrupt your sleep, though. Write it down with a set time for when you will tackle the problem productively in the morning. Then go to sleep knowing that you've scheduled a time to worry about it and therefore don't need to do it at 4 a.m.!

- If anxiety is an ongoing problem, you might like to incorporate a calming cup of herbal tea to relax you, combine a calming nighttime meditation ritual with your journaling, or use soothing lights, music, and gentle stretching to encourage your mind to calm down. Talking to a counsellor or therapist may be necessary in the long run

All that said, nighttime reflection doesn't have to be ultra-structured. You've spent the whole day in an active, busy mode; now's the time to "rest and digest." Trust that your unconscious mind will slowly start to work through the day's problems, and be still for a while so that ideas can gently rise to the surface.

Quiet time when you're doing "nothing" can sometimes be the best thing in the evenings. This is often when we rest, heal, or have new insights into problems and situations. If you *don't* take the time to deliberately decompress your mind this way, you'll be going to bed still wired and buzzing, which will naturally lead to fitful sleep, bad dreams, or insomnia. So, give yourself the gift of an evening reflection ritual.

Tip 16: Prepare for the Day Ahead

As we've seen, good nighttime routines go hand in hand with good morning routines. You wake up with the same mindset as the one you went to sleep with, so it's worth going to sleep on the right side of the bed! Part of putting the day passed to bed, so to speak, is to plan for the next day. This could mean:

- Setting your alarms
- Getting your day's outfit lined up and ready so you can just shower and get dressed in the morning
- Charging your phone
- Packing lunches, freezing water bottles, or putting things that you need to take to work by the door so you're ready to grab them and go
- If you can, outline a rough to-do list and prioritize your most important tasks. It's a good idea to know exactly what your most important task is (or the three most important at a maximum) so you can start with them when you're fresh and have the most energy

94

- Make sure you won't be waking up to chaos. For example, tidy up the kitchen the night before so you aren't faced with dirty dishes first thing in the morning

As with other habits we've discussed, you want to make your evening routines as automatic and easy as possible. The reason is that at night, you're tired. Your resources for the day are probably depleted or close to empty—you simply don't have the wherewithal to do any mental heavy lifting. So it shouldn't be a mad dash to complete everything to prepare for the next day, but rather something you do as seamlessly and effortlessly as you brush your teeth in the evening.

Don't make any major life changes or big plans in the evening, but do make sure you're paving the way for a smooth launch the next morning. If you're too tried to tackle an issue at night, schedule a moment the next day where you'll look more closely at it. Don't be a hero and think that you're saving time by doing *everything* the night before . . . you might just end up stressing yourself needlessly. Avoid:

- You guessed it—phones and glowing pixelated screens play havoc with your natural circadian rhythms and frazzle your nerves. If you do plan and schedule, do it briefly with paper and pen
- Marathon TV sessions. Set an evening TV budget and then *physically get up* off the couch when a show ends to tell yourself to transition to the next activity
- Switch devices to eye-friendly, non-blue light in the evenings, or consider installing apps that turn devices off after a certain time
- Keep work, devices, or study materials out of the bedroom. Keep it a serene haven away from the troubles of the world!
- If you find yourself ruminating over the day ahead and can't get to sleep—get up and sit elsewhere for a while to avoid forming a negative association of sleeplessness with

your bed. Go somewhere dimly lit and quiet and listen to a gentle podcast till you feel sleepy, then try again

Sometimes, preparing for the day ahead is nothing more complicated than taking a deep breath and saying to yourself, "This day is finished. I did my best. Now I'm resting tonight, and tomorrow is another day." Use little rituals to put the old day to rest and hold off the new day until you're rested and ready to face it. You can light candles, do a daily guided meditation or visualization, or even tell yourself out loud, "The past is the past. The future hasn't happened yet. Right now, my only job is to sleep deeply."

Tip 17: Renew Your Commitment

As you're writing notes in your journal, you may find yourself naturally arriving back at your main goals. Sometimes, in the fluster and busyness of the day, we can lose a little of our focus and determination. We get tired as the hours wear on and forget that passion and drive that originally made us commit to making changes. In the peace and quiet of the evening, it's time to renew and refresh that commitment you originally made for yourself.

As you sleep, the cells of your tissues and organs are all regenerating, healing, and cleaning themselves. Your brain is working hard to process the day's sensory data and make sense of it, consolidating memories and working through everything that it's learned. Your immune system resets, your breath and heart rate slow, and your body goes into renewal mode. You can do the same thing for your commitment: renew it.

Did you face something especially challenging today? Acknowledge that and give yourself space to recuperate, adjust, and know you can start again with it tomorrow. You'll be tired, but pause to give yourself time to regather your mental resources and remind yourself of what actually matters. Do any boundaries need tightening? Any developing habits need a closer look? Tap into your original WHY—

your reason for wanting change—and remember the journey you're on.

Whether you're trying to lose weight, exercise more, or just be healthier in general, zoom out and look at where you are on your path. Reconnect to those values and principles that inspire you. As you sleep, let your enthusiasm fill up again, and let your strength and determination refresh itself. Read a little motivational material or your favorite inspirational quotes. Go through your personal manifesto or meditate for a few moments on what you're trying to achieve and why. Tell yourself you can do it. Better yet—that you *are* doing it right now.

Visualize yourself waking up tomorrow morning, full of vigor and focused determination, ready as ever to carry on with your journey. When paired with an acknowledgment of how far you've already come, this is a deeply satisfying way to finish the day. You'll feel content, accomplished, fortified, and inspired to carry on. Sweet dreams!

Summary:

- A night routine consolidates and closes off the day, giving you time to check in on yourself and prepare for the next day. Your night routine influences the quality of your sleep that night, which in turn influences the following day. Thus, night routines and morning routines go hand in hand to create a structured, productive, and healthy lifestyle.
- At night, focus on winding down, relaxing, and coming to an awareness of yourself and what's happened throughout the day. As with morning routines, make a small change, give it time, observe and tweak, then make another small change.
- Make your most impactful changes first. For most people, this means going to bed earlier and getting more (and better quality) sleep. Start with sleeping at the same time every night and see if there are any weak spots in your sleep hygiene.

- After a day of activity, pull back and enjoy quiet, gentle time alone. Reflect, journal, appraise the day past, and let things settle and digest.
- Plan the day ahead so you are ready to go first thing in the morning. It's easier to relax into deep sleep when you are confident that you're prepared to face the new day.
- Take a moment to remind yourself of why you're changing, and see how far you've come on your journey. Renew your commitment to yourself, refresh your willpower, and give yourself a pat on the back for all you've achieved.

Chapter 5: Overcoming Bad Days

Two things are true when you're trying to make a lifestyle change:

1. You can do it. **It is possible**. Others just like you have done it, and you will too if you set your mind to it.
2. There will be challenges. There will be setbacks. There will be bad days. Guaranteed!

No plan to succeed would go very far without a plan for how to manage the inevitable setbacks. And those setbacks really are inevitable. Are you going to face these obstacles with utter surprise and disappointment or are you going to be prepared and ready to overcome them regardless?

What if You Want to Give Up?

It's normal to want to give up. Change is hard, and there's a good reason you've stayed so long in your comfort zone—it's comfortable! That means striving to be better can be *uncomfortable*. This isn't a sign that anything is wrong or that you have to stop. It's just a sign that you're changing, pushing your boundaries, and working hard.

We've spoken a lot about positive mindset, but your attitude to "failure" is just as important in defining your outcome. You will slip up eventually; the only variable is how you will respond to it. Firstly, don't see it as failure at all. Pigging out one day when you promised you'd eat better or skipping a few workouts aren't the end of the world. It's data. Instead of going into judgment mode and wallowing in self-hate or self-pity (or worse, giving up entirely), become curious about why you slipped up and what you can learn for next time round.

Were your expectations too high and did you try to make quantum leaps when baby steps would have been better?
Did you put yourself in temptation's way?
Were you tired, stressed, or overwhelmed?

What to Do if you Fall off the Wagon

If you fall off the wagon, stop, take a deep breath, and relax. First things first, don't make things worse. By this I mean don't take a small mistake as permission to make a bigger mistake. You gobbled up something unhealthy? Fine. But don't despair and decide that you might as well carry on bingeing now that you've already come this far.

You've become conscious of the error; that's a start, well done. The next step is, as soon as you possibly can, make a single, conscious decision to act concretely in the right direction. This doesn't have to be big. It just has to be a real world refreshing of your commitment. Digging down this way can break the spell of self-pity or excuse making and focus your attention where it matters: how can you get back on the path?

The third step, once you've taken that action, is to completely forget about the slip-up. Seriously. If you've learned what you can and adjusted accordingly, if you've taken a step in the right direction again, then just let the mistake go. It won't help you one bit to hold on to it in guilt or shame. Use the courage of being back on the wagon already to forgive yourself for having temporarily fallen off it!

You're Not Seeing Results—Now What?

It might be that you don't have a full-blown mistake, but rather creep to a place where you're seriously doubting the point of carrying on. Maybe you've been diligently following your diet and exercise plan for weeks and the weight is dropping so painfully slowly that you barely notice it— or worse, you've gained a little. What then?

As you can imagine, your first task is to stay wide awake and conscious. Zoom in on what you feel. Double check your manifesto, your values and principles, your original reasons, and your ultimate goal. Spend a moment in contemplation and become curious about this new obstacle in your way. Often, feeling discouraged with not seeing results quickly enough is a sign of:

- Unrealistic expectations
- Impatience
- Fear of change

Ask honestly if you're expecting miracles overnight. Losing weight, building muscle, or making big lifestyle changes take time— more time than you might think. Have you perhaps been expecting that you'll quickly reach your goal and then get to relax and celebrate? The truth is, with ongoing lifestyle change, there is no glamorous "after" photo, no perfect day when all your problems are solved and you don't have to work hard anymore. Expecting this, even unconsciously, can make us impatient.

On the other hand, you might be playing with the idea of quitting precisely because you're afraid of succeeding. The prospect of putting yourself out there, of expecting more, of being responsible for your life, of taking risks . . . these things can be scary, and people can jeopardize themselves and choose to stay as they are, as unfulfilling as that may be. If you're having problems like this, revisit your goals and your timeline and get honest about what you can expect. Break your tasks down into smaller steps and don't forget to acknowledge and celebrate smaller milestones on the way— they're imperative for keeping you motivated!

Tip 18: Use Creativity to Your Advantage

When you find yourself in the middle of a bad day, don't freak out. Get curious and find creative ways to bend around it. You're sick and can't work out except for gentle walking? Well, then do gentle walking!

Here's a tip: temptation and the desire to quit actually come with a built-in warning bell, and that warning bell is boredom. If you notice yourself getting bored, take this as a sign that you're not far away from making excuses, procrastinating, or cheating on your plan. Step in the moment you notice you're bored and take action by switching things up and reminding yourself of your original commitment. Take a moment to reconnect to your inspiration and refresh your promise to yourself, and then get creative to banish that boredom. What do I mean by get creative? Well, the only limit is your imagination:

- Try a different workout, or do the same workout in a different location. Up the intensity, add a wild card element, or give yourself an extra, fun challenge like skipping that day's workout and doing an intense hour-long salsa class instead

- On your daily walk, go a different route, try the same route with ankle weights, or experiment with doing sprints in that field you always walk past. Climb a tree!

- If your diet is boring you, challenge yourself to cook something novel that sticks to the rules. Try new fruit and veggies or novel combinations. Or, eat outside for an impromptu picnic
- Mix up your rewards. Make a deal with yourself that you'll do something really new and exciting once you complete a mini-milestone
- Bring a little fun into things. You don't *have to* sit through boring, chore-like workouts. Include more heart-pumping and feel-good dance classes, sports, or even just playing with your kids (no kids? Great—you get to be the kid!). If you're feeling uninspired, get outdoors and do some good honest manual labor— intense DIY or gardening are great for the soul, as is a home declutter or spring clean

Bringing creativity into your daily routine is about seeing obstacles and, instead of shrugging your shoulders and concluding that you can't go forward, become curious and ask, "**How** can I go forward? What will I have to change to overcome this?" Remember, you're in charge. If something isn't working, don't throw in the towel and give up. Change it *until it works*. Many people think that they can't make drastic changes to their health because they hate the gym or can't afford it, and they can't picture themselves eating ridiculous "health food." But who says you have to go to the gym? Who says you have to eat kale? (Go ahead, I officially give you permission not to eat kale if you don't want to!)

It's worth remembering that improving your health and wellbeing is not meant to be a punishment. It's not work. It's something wonderful you're giving yourself because you're worth the effort. That means you don't have to force yourself through a meager and tasteless dinner of salmon and steamed broccoli every single evening. "No pain no gain" is a maxim that emphasizes that you need to work hard to see results. But it doesn't mean that living a healthy lifestyle is supposed to feel awful and boring—after all, doesn't thinking this way simply make it more likely that you go straight back to how you were? It all comes down to mindset. Your "hard work" may actually be in challenging the assumptions you have about what healthy people do every day.

If you're finding that resistance is coming up, or that you're tempted to give up or make excuses, make a deal with yourself: agree that you *can* throw in the towel if you really want to . . . but first, you have to at least try again with a few changes before giving up completely. More often than not, you'll find that shaking things up with a little creative thinking is all that's needed to get your momentum back and overcome that roadblock.

Tip 19: Find Your Well of Inspiration

Let's be honest here. You already *know* what you ought to be doing. You *know* intellectually that it's good to eat your veggies, drink lots of water, and exercise daily. It's not about mentally comprehending the need for a healthy lifestyle, though; it's about motivating yourself to actually do it.

Your inspiration and motivation are like a power source—if you don't have one or you're not tapping into it regularly, you're going to find your enthusiasm flagging often. On the other hand, if you know how to amp yourself up when it matters, you'll be able to fuel yourself for the long, hard journey to where you want to be.

We've already seen how important it is to have a goal, to be dedicated to that goal, and to maintain your focus and positive mentality by smart, daily routines morning and night. But sometimes (especially on really bad days), you're going to need to know how to bring out the big guns and inspire yourself back on to the path.

There's a disconnect—when you start out on your mission, you're full of vigor and enthusiasm. You can see the end point in crystal clarity, and you want it so badly you can taste it. But fast forward a few months where you're stuck in the muck of it and having a hard day, perhaps even taking a few steps backward—then what? Where did all your enthusiasm go?

Enthusiasm, motivation, and zest are like a deep well you can draw from to keep you going on your journey. But it's up to you to know where that well is, to know how to access it, and even to know how to top it off when necessary. Somewhere in the future, you will find yourself looking at your goals, at your choices, hell—even at this book— and thinking it's all useless. You'll be at that fork in the road where you can choose to push forward (difficult) or fall back on the same old bad behavior (easy). If you're in this situation, take it as another warning sign—your inspiration tank is desperately low! Here's how to fill it back up again:

- Have a pre-saved collection of truly inspirational videos or podcasts to listen to every time you're feeling uninspired or weak willed. Other people's enthusiasm can be contagious!

- Make a playlist of inspiring music . . . there has got to be at least a few songs that set your soul on fire and remind you of what's possible
- An unusual thing to do is compile an "inspiration folder" where you collect things that make you feel proud of yourself and your accomplishments. Fill it with praise from others and compliments, pictures where you looked good, lists of your achievements, your personal manifesto and value statement, or even certificates and accolades you've achieved. Look at themes and remember what you achieved—even though you went through tough patches, just as you are going through one now
- Collect a book of inspirational quotes, poems, articles, or even song lyrics that speak to you
- Find and enjoy motivational artwork that taps right down into your deepest motivation. Sometimes, seeing beautiful things beyond everyday ordinary limitations can

stir that creativity and energy within you—what do you want to contribute? What do you want your life to stand for ultimately?

- Remind yourself of your Big Why, which is your deep motivational powerhouse. For example, you may be wanting to lose weight not for vanity, but because you want to be fit and healthy and be around for your kids rather than die of heart disease by age sixty. You might choose to look at their pictures and visualize yourself being their hero by showing them that reaching your dreams is possible

- Read stories of people who have overcome challenges—nothing gets you back on the horse as much as knowing that other people have worked miracles with far less adversity than you are currently facing!

Tip 20: Be Accountable

Being inspired is a power source that comes from within, but there are external sources of motivation, too. Peer pressure is certainly one of them, but you can use the power of social encouragement in a much less damaging way. Being accountable is a little like asking others to bear some of the burden of responsibility. Think of it as distributing the duty a little!

Being accountable to another person is a great way to prepare yourself for those inevitable difficult days or slip-ups. Though you might be able to convince yourself that you really absolutely couldn't do what you promised you would, you might get a reality check and feel a little embarrassed making that same argument to someone else. You can leverage this power of not wanting to let others down (or, let's face it, be slightly humiliated to go back on your word!). True, it's not the intrinsic motivation that's most associated with meeting your own goals, but it will get the job done in a pinch. It will help you overcome the bump in the road so you can carry on and find your own inner motivation a little later when you're stronger.

Being accountable to someone else, or indeed something else, is not difficult to set up. As with all other approaches and tips we've already discussed for dealing with bad days, the trick is in the preparation.

- Ask a friend or family member to check in with you to see if you've done your workout or followed through on your eating plan. Even better if that person is also trying to improve their health as well—you can mutually support one another. Check in with them by dropping them a message or even sending them a selfie of you in the gym!
- If it works with your personality (it won't work for everyone), build in a little competition. See who does the most steps every day or every week, for example. The point is not to fight for prizes or be mean to each other, but to replace excuses with genuine effort to be as good as you can

- If you can afford it and like the idea, get a professional involved; for example, a personal trainer, nutritionist, or even a mental health professional. A life coach or similar can take you to task when you start sprouting excuses. They can believe in you on those days you don't quite believe in yourself

- Announce your goals. Don't go overboard, but sometimes telling someone outright, "I'm going to do this marathon in two months' time," is a powerful way to set it in stone in your own mind. You might feel lazy and uncommitted to training some days, but tough. You said you would, so do it.

- Share success. This is a gentler approach, but keeping others appraised of where you are on your journey ropes them in and makes you more accountable. You'll feel like they're watching and rooting for you, and this makes you want to do better on those difficult days. It's not a question of shame or guilt, but rather realizing that you have the opportunity to impress and inspire others or make them proud

- If you really want to go all out with accountability, get a trusted friend and literally sign a contract with them, binding you to your promise. Get creative: you could make a deal with a close friend where you agree to pay them twenty dollars every workout you skip. It's the nuclear option, but it will work!

Again, the best time to factor in some accountability is before you need it. This is why it's so important to anticipate failure and plan accordingly. The thing you want to avoid is being alone with all your laziness and excuses and no outside observers to catch you or remind you of what you were trying to achieve.

Tip 21: Clean Up Your Mindset

A bad day can mean that you've failed to prepare, or that you're overtired, or that you're simply human and mess up sometimes. But a bad day can also be a sign that your attitude needs a tweak.

While you're working hard to change your body, don't forget that the hardest thing to change can be the mind. Your body right now, and all your daily habits and routines, are a reflection of what goes on between your ears. If you want to change your life, you need to change all the beliefs that created that life in the first place. This means getting real about your "personal narratives" and the self-talk playing in your mind all day every day.

If you've fallen off the wagon, it's a good time to check in with your overall mindset and see if you can identify any self-sabotaging beliefs and thoughts. Sometimes you might need to completely overhaul your perspective, and other times, it's more a question of gently rebalancing your focus and fine-tuning yourself back to your priorities.

You could pay someone hundreds of dollars to help you with Cognitive Behavioral

Therapy, (this is an excellent option if you go down that path), but you can also make significant changes all on your own right now, today. It's a simple two-step process: identifying disempowering beliefs that are holding you back and then adjusting or changing them into something that will support your evolution.

I say it's simple, but that doesn't mean it's easy. Reworking your core beliefs takes time, honesty, and courage. But it's the most rewarding work you'll probably ever do. Here's a (very brief) outline for how to do run a mindset diagnostic on yourself when you're having a hard time sticking to your commitments.

Step 1: Without thinking too hard about it, scribble down some beliefs and feelings that come to mind when you consider the challenges you're facing. Maybe you write things like, "I'm not cut out for this" or "I'm a loser" or "I didn't do it perfectly so I might as well give up." Once you put some ideas down, dig deeper into each. Take time to flesh each idea out without judgment.

Step 2: Take some time to condense the ideas into themes, and then look at these core beliefs. What effect do they have on your life? Do they inspire you to be better or do they make you hate yourself? Do they encourage you to be the best you can be or do they help you stay small? Finally, ask who you would be *without* these thoughts and beliefs.

Step 3: Gently adjust the beliefs. If you have been telling yourself that you need to be perfect all the time to be a worthwhile human being, rewrite that core belief into "I am imperfect and that's okay." Look for extreme, all-or-nothing statements and mellow them out a bit. "I always fail" becomes "I've failed now, and that's okay. It doesn't mean I can't succeed next time."

So many of us desperately try to improve our lives while all the while carrying deep-down beliefs about ourselves that basically believe it's impossible. We feel that we don't really deserve good things, or that we will never really aspire to much. Success is for other people and not us. We feel that we are not up to the challenge and fear being disappointed, or we tell ourselves that discomfort and uncertainty on the path means we're doing something wrong.

The range of core beliefs is infinite—nobody can tell you what yours are. It's up to you to look within, identify the "programming" you're running on, and decide whether it's really working for you. If not, change it.

- Keep your ears pricked for words like always, never, everyone, nothing—they're a sign of unhelpful, inaccurate core beliefs and black-and-white thinking
- Notice the content of thoughts and beliefs, but also how they make you feel. Are you talking to yourself in a way that leaves you feeling ashamed and paralyzed? Would you say to a loved one what you say to yourself?
- Refuse to take your word for it. When you hear a familiar core belief, ask yourself if you have any actual

124

evidence for it being true (hint: you usually don't)

Tip 22: Make Friends with Discomfort—and Prepare for It

Let's say you're on a diet and doing your best to eat less and eat more nutritious, healthy food. Sounds great, but now it's an hour after lunch and you're *ravenous*. You're in the danger zone and at risk of dropping your commitment, especially if one of your core beliefs is "I shouldn't have to be uncomfortable."

The big boring truth? Change is uncomfortable. Losing weight means eating less, and that inevitably comes with hunger and not being able to eat everything you want. Getting into shape takes effort and sometimes leaves you sore the next day. We return to the idea of expecting setbacks and being prepared for them. We need to realize that a certain amount of discomfort is built into the change process. *Overall*, we have a net gain to our wellbeing, but there will still be moments along that journey that feel decidedly worse than where we've come from.

Discomfort isn't a sign that anything is wrong, or a reason to give up. It's not something you can't handle. It'll pass. Gnawing hunger, cravings for junk food—they'll pass. Tired and sore muscles? They'll pass too. If you can embrace the fact that you will be hungry or sore or tired at some point, you can begin to see it as positive evidence that you are making progress. It's proof that you're working right at the boundaries of your comfort zone and getting better. That's something to celebrate!

As always, anticipate and come prepared:

- If you're really hungry, make sure you have a bunch of healthy but low calorie snacks at hand to curb the craving—fresh berries, carrot and celery sticks, salted rice cakes, salads, or fruit can tide you over till your next meal

- If you can, just sit with your hunger. Become mindful. It's uncomfortable, yes, but is it really all that bad? Can you notice that your cravings actually disappear if you can just ride them out for a few minutes?
- Distract yourself. Often what feels like hunger is just boredom. Get busy and you won't notice that you're hungry
- Alternatively, your feeling of hunger can also be simply thirst. Stay hydrated or indulge in a nice cup of tea or a cool drink. Obviously, avoid sugar-laden or calorific drinks
- Avoid extra temptations that will only exacerbate your feelings of lack—for example, stay away from junk food aisles in the grocery store and give yourself enough time to prepare healthy home-cooked meals so you're not tempted to get something easy and unhealthy
- If you're feeling achy after a workout, invest in some magnesium salts to bathe in to help you recover. Some

gentle yoga and stretching can help soothe hardworking muscles, too

- If you're finding a particular workout or activity challenging, it's okay to find alternative ways through it. Take a breather, try a simplified move, or simply go more slowly. As long as you're genuinely challenging yourself, don't worry about keeping up with others or achieving impressive feats

Finally, it's worth mentioning a particular kind of discomfort that you won't see mentioned in many self-help books: the discomfort that comes after a binge, a skipped workout, or a failure to step up to your commitments. As we've seen, forgiveness and quick, beneficial action are the best solutions for getting sidetracked off your path. Tell yourself: *Making mistakes is okay. Feeling bad about messing up will pass. I can have a sense of humor about it, and some self-compassion. Feeling bad right now is not the end of the world. It's not something I can't handle or move on from.*

Summary:

- Change is always possible, but obstacles, setbacks, and failure are a given. To make successful changes, you need to anticipate and prepare for these setbacks.

- Be mindful of when you feel like giving up, and try to act as early as possible to adjust, take a rest, or find a creative way around the problem. If you mess up, the key is to ask what you can learn from the mistake, then immediately commit to action that puts you back on the path again. Forgive yourself and move on, empowered to do better next time.

- If you're getting impatient or demoralized, you may need to have more frequent milestones or rewards, or else re-evaluate your expectations.

- On bad days, instead of giving up, try to mix things up instead. Novelty and creativity can get momentum going again.

- Make sure you know where to find a renewable source of inspiration; tap into motivational quotes, podcasts, books, etc. to keep you inspired.

- Don't go it alone—find accountability with others.

- If you're having a very hard time, it may be worth having a closer look at your mindset, your core beliefs, your expectations, or the way you're framing your goals. Remind yourself that change is possible—your job is simply to find out how it's possible.

- Finally, make friends with discomfort and uncertainty. Getting out of your comfort zone is hard, but it's where change happens!

Chapter 6: Reaching Milestones

Kinds of Goals to Set for Yourself

The recurring themes of this book? Reaching your goals takes strategic determination, consistency, and patience.

But now let's turn to the question of the goals you should be aiming for in the first place. All of our efforts—setting up good morning and evening routines, having contingency plans for obstacles, fine-tuning your mindset—all of them are in service of the big prize at the end, our goals. It's not something you might have given too much thought, but the quality of your goals makes a huge difference to your ability to achieve them.

People can waste time working toward an outcome that they actually realize was unimportant once they achieve it. Or, once started, they see that they've bitten off way more than they can chew. Right now, you have a desire: to be healthier. And you know that you need to make changes to get there. The way you frame your goals forms the paving stones covering the distance from where you are now to where you desire to be. Effective goals are what are called SMART goals:

S – specific
M – measurable
A – achievable
R – realistic
T – time bound

So, a good goal is, "I want to eat five servings of fruit and veggies every day in the upcoming month."
A bad goal is, "I want to watch my diet a bit more closely," or, "I want to be more fit."

Why is Goal Setting Important?

If you set a vague, wishy-washy, or unrealistic goal, you simply won't reach it. Then, you'll have wasted time, gotten nowhere, *and* demoralized yourself in the process. So far, we've discussed strategies and approaches for making your dreams come true . . . but none of that means much unless we have a clear, focused vision of what that dream is and why we want to achieve it.

Even if your goals are SMART goals, they still need to be right for you personally, and speak to your values in some way. Unless you are explicit and detailed with your goals, you might not notice that they are not really making you a better person or helping you build the life you really want for yourself.

It may seem odd to end the book with a discussion of goals, but when you think about it, this is exactly where we find them in real life—at the end of our journeys.

How to Celebrate Once You've Reached a Milestone

What should you do once you've actually achieved a goal? Whether it's a small daily milestone or a culmination of years' worth of effort, the answer is obvious: celebrate! We've seen why it's important to acknowledge and mark your progress through observing your goals as you go. Feeling proud and accomplished keeps you motivated and positive. Nothing in the world compares to the feeling of knowing that you set your mind to something, worked hard, and achieved it.

This is a truly joyful, exciting moment. You are confirming all at once that yes, you *can* do it—and did! You are telling yourself that you are worth the effort, that you are capable and competent, and that you have earned the right to claim some new characteristics—those of discipline, determination, and courage. Well done to you!

The prospect of this satisfaction, of this reward, is what might power you on your difficult days when you want to give up. Knowing that the alternative is a loss of faith in yourself, disappointment, and even shame, hard work suddenly doesn't seem like such a high price to pay for feeling so good about yourself instead. Think of motivation as envy for your future self— look at how amazingly proud and satisfied you're going to be in the future, and let your present self step up to the plate to bring you closer to that vision.

Don't you look so good in that fulfilled state? A funny thing happens when people achieve the goals they set for themselves— they suddenly get inspired to set even more! They wonder, "Why didn't I push myself to do this sooner?" Think about that. Not only do they not feel like they pushed themselves too far or that the goal was beyond them, but rather that they can suddenly see limitless potential for themselves, and now trust their ability to actually claim the things they want.

It's powerful stuff. And it's available to you. Many people fail to recognize opportunity, as the saying goes, because it first appears to them as hard work. But this state of blissful and happy achievement is open and available to you. The path to victory is not mysterious or exclusive . . . it's laid out plainly for you. All you have to do is walk it. One step at a time.

Once you reach a goal, you have one of the most wonderful gifts of all: the understanding that life is actually *continual improvement*. It dawns on you that the goal isn't the prize at all. Fulfilling your inbuilt potential and having the opportunity to go even further still—that's the real gift.

Tip 23: Make Use of Time Limits

Okay. Let's come back to earth for a moment. Big goals have a simple anatomy: they're made up of smaller goals. And the way you make smaller goals is to set a time limit on yourself for achieving a certain outcome. This is the "T" part of the SMART acronym, and though it's on the end, it may be the most important criterion. There are several reasons for putting a deadline on yourself:

- You're more likely to actually get it done, i.e. your focus is narrowed and you're on the clock, so to speak
- You're less likely to get overwhelmed—losing a pound a week seems less intimidating than losing almost fifty pounds in a year, although it's the same amount
- You give yourself the opportunity to course correct along the way. By appraising your progress, you can adjust and fine tune, making yourself more efficient

Perhaps most importantly, when you put a timer on your goals, you hold yourself accountable. You may say, "I want to lose weight," but then immediately follow it with that famous, self-sabotaging word: "someday." When this word pops up, what it really means is "never." When you put a fixed deadline on yourself, though, what you're doing is taking your own word for it.

You are committing to yourself by not settling for a weak "someday." People who fail to nail down their goals to a real point in the future may secretly not have much belief in themselves that it will ever really happen. Are you unconsciously limiting yourself this way?

What does a time-limited goal look like? You could set a deadline for yourself, which is a point at which you stop and appraise how far you've come and whether you've achieved your aims. (See why it's so important to have SMART goals? Unless your goals are "measurable," you won't have a way to determine whether you've actually achieved them or not!)

For example, you could say that by March 25th, you will be able to run five miles. Time-limited goals can be of any length, from making a promise about what you'll achieve in the next few minutes, to where you plan to be in a year's time. Preferably, you have several goals at once, with a mix of short, medium, and long term. The short-term goals are like the intermediate stations on the train tracks that you stop and call at on your journey—the long-term goal is your final destination.

A few things can happen once the deadline arrives, and this will determine how you respond and move forward.

- **Reached your goal?** Great! Was it too easy, and could you ramp it up for next time? Think about the next step in the journey and how to apply what you've learned already for the next stage of your development. Reward yourself, celebrate, and most importantly, update your inner sense of identity—you *are* a person who can change and improve!

- **Reached your goal but only partially?** Go into detective mode and become curious about why that is. Go through the SMART criteria and see if the goal was maybe unrealistic, too hard, irrelevant, or too vague. Did you run out of time? Look closely at what stopped you from reaching your goal and then make concrete plans to remove it. Remember that the problem might not be you and a lack of discipline, but also a poorly formulated goal. Have you made *any* advances? Focus on how you did so, then try to do more of the same.

- **Failed to reach your goal?** There's a reason for that, and it's your job to find it out. No, failing to achieve a goal doesn't mean you can give up or berate yourself or conclude that change is impossible. Go back to the drawing board and be super honest with yourself—where is the problem? Without judgment, see where you can improve in your process and commit to taking one concrete step to do better. It's important not to carry on doing the same old thing—you'll only fail again in precisely the same way.

You may discover that you have neglected your daily routines, or that you are undermining yourself with a negative mindset. Or you may find that actually, you underestimate yourself and can do much, much more—set a bigger goal! Or you might discover that it's time for a different approach—maybe you need more accountability, more time for reflection, more baby steps or a more reliable source of inspiration. You can only gain this insight if you have time-limited goals. Without them, you bumble along, never giving yourself the chance to *learn*.

Tip 24: Splurge!

Look, I get it. All this talk of discipline and dedication and laser focus can all seem a bit . . . serious. But a big part of a winning mindset is to realize that self-improvement and growth are supposed to be fun. It's meant to feel light, inspiring, and doable. Too many people have a sense of doom when they think of diet and exercise. They picture themselves marching into a figurative sweat shop where it's all work and no play, steamed veggies for dinner and an early bedtime. In other words, it sounds like hell!

But if you entertain a perspective where living well is seen as some sort of suffering, what incentive do you have to keep up with it? The very second you reach a small goal, you'll think, "Thank God! Now I'm allowed to quit and get on with normal living again!" But the mistake is to think that a healthy lifestyle is somehow not normal living. That it's a temporary punishment that you endure only to get the rewards, and once you do, you grab them and run away back to your Netflix binges and junk food. I don't need to tell you, though, where this mindset leads!

A big part of reaching and celebrating milestones is giving yourself a nice, big, fat reward.

But, you need to be careful here. You don't want to teach yourself that living unhealthily is a reward for temporarily living in denial and deprivation. If you reach your healthy eating goal and reward yourself with an ice cream, what are you really communicating to yourself? Is this message one that will help you sustain your long-term goals or undermine them?

Let me be clear: you deserve to enjoy your life. Living well, eating healthily, moving your body, and reaching your fitness goal is a joy and a privilege and a real gift. It's there for you to relish. But, it's never *health vs. happiness*. You can have both! Rather than rewarding yourself with the very things you are trying to move away from, rethink the concept of reward entirely. What you want is to create a lifestyle that is so good, normal, healthy, and comfortable that *you don't want or need a reward*—simply living that way is satisfying enough. Big difference, huh?

Consider two examples. Jane is trying to lose thirty pounds and feel better about herself.

Scenario 1: She goes on a punishingly restrictive diet for a month and over-exercises until she's half dead. She works so hard, in fact, that when she loses ten pounds that month, she feels she truly deserves a "treat." She buys a tub of ice cream on the way home. Feeling mentally and physically deprived for so long, her treat quickly turns into a full-on binge. She spirals into self-hate and despair, and in a week, she is depressed, bloated, and twelve pounds heavier than before.

Scenario 2: She adopts a moderate diet and exercise plan she knows she can maintain for the long term. She notices with pride that she has lost five pounds after a month. She loves feeling a little lighter, a little more in control, a little more vibrant, and full of energy. She occasionally gets cravings for ice cream, and when she does, she gives herself a little with no judgment. But she also decides that she loves fresh blueberries and commits to making this her treat— aren't they just as good, really? At the end of six months, she's lost more than thirty pounds and is still going strong. She eats blueberries *and* ice cream, both in moderation. The end.

When you reach your goal, go ahead— splurge! It's okay to enjoy life! But it's a smarter strategy to start looking for joy and bliss on the everyday path you're on. Focus on how good you feel after a modest, healthy meal. Notice that your "treat" is seldom worth the bad feelings. Notice how doing the right thing often does feel pretty good. When you crave a treat or a night off, enjoy it. No guilt. No need to freak out—you can be a healthy person who still has wiggle room in life to let your hair down occasionally. You're not a professional bodybuilder . . . if you consistently make the right choice eighty percent of the time? That's enough.

Tip 25: Update Your Self-image

Remember the chapter on mindset? And all the ways our inner narratives and core beliefs can either help or hinder our attempts to improve? Well, once you reach a goal, you need to do something important: adjust your inner sense of who you are now that you have, in fact, changed.

It's a little like losing weight and then ceremonially throwing away trousers that are now too big for you. There are, of course, *mental trousers* that we may still carry on wearing internally. It can take time for our internal conception of ourselves to catch up with the real, concrete changes we've made for ourselves. Making this psychological update is important because if you still feel and think and behave as the person you were, you may still make choices that reflect a less evolved version of yourself. You could sabotage your success or even reverse it.

When you congratulate yourself for reaching a goal (yes, even and maybe especially a tiny goal), you are also experiencing what it's like to be someone new—the kind of person who does that kind of thing. All those stories about how you can't and how it's difficult and how you'll never get there? Turns out those stories aren't true, and you *are* in fact a healthy, disciplined person. After a goal is achieved, take a moment to actually let that sink in: you are that person.

How do we update our internal image so it lines up with the outer one?

- **Watch your language**. Instead of saying, "I'm *trying* to do XYZ," say, "I'm doing XYZ." Don't frame your efforts as a one-time freak event, don't put yourself down or minimize your achievements, and don't assume that making impressive changes is for other people and not for you. Let your language reflect that you already believe in yourself

- **Walk the walk**. You are not an imposter. You're achieving your dreams, so act like it! Carry yourself as though you expect to succeed

- **Think about who you are**. Now might be the time to rewrite old scripts and reconsider who you've always felt you are. In the same way as cognitive behavioral therapy allows us to examine and gently adjust our thoughts, we can also look at our identity and ask, is this really me? Is this who I am and who I want to be? It can be completely empowering and liberating to realize that not only can you change this, but that you are already in the process

As an example of adjusting one's identity, consider Mike, who for a long time wanted to adopt a vegan diet. It fit his principles, and he also yearned for a healthier, plant-based life. But he had spent so long saying things like, "I'd love to be a vegan but oh man, I could never give up cheese!" and, "You have to be super ultra-disciplined to be a vegan, I guess."

After successfully eating a vegan diet for a week, Mike pauses to reflect and notices himself saying some version of the above to friends. But then, he wonders, is this vision of himself still relevant? He might have seen himself in the past as an unfixable cheese-addict and the opposite of whatever "super ultra-disciplined" is, but then, here was conflicting evidence: he had in fact been a vegan for a week. Couldn't he do the same again and be a vegan for two weeks? Looking honestly at his thoughts and beliefs about his identity, he realized he had outgrown his old idea of who he was. He wasn't a person trying to be a vegan. He was one.

To have belief in yourself, you sometimes need to change your idea of what that "self" is. Do you continue to think of yourself as fat, lazy, too old, too weak, too far gone to improve? Do you still characterize yourself as someone who can't really change, or won't? Once you reach a goal, absorb it. Let it sink in and settle. Allow yourself to expand and become bigger. You've done all the hard work of achieving change—now claim it!

Tip 26: Keep Your Focus

Focus, as we know, is important. Don't set so many goals that you can't keep up or that force you to dilute your attention. Pace yourself and have a good balance between effort and reward, work and the recognition of that work.

One good strategy is to have one goal per day. For example, Monday's goal can be to walk ten thousand steps. Tuesday can be doing two hundred jumping jacks. Wednesday can be drinking one gallon of water. In the very beginning, your mini-goals will take some time to achieve, but after a while, you should start to find it easier and easier to tick them off the list. Once this happens, that's your cue to ramp up the intensity. You can do this by giving yourself a bigger goal to reach (e.g. walking eleven thousand steps) or changing the time limit (e.g. doing those two hundred jumping jacks, but faster). You could also set a new, broader goal—to maintain an unbroken string of smaller goals; for example, you drink a gallon of water every day for a solid month. These are just examples—how you ramp up your goals depends entirely on you and what you're ultimately trying to achieve.

Look at it this way: maintaining focus is a question of knowing at all times exactly what goal you are working toward. Don't be without a goal, but at the same time, don't have so many hanging over you that you feel overwhelmed or confused. You need to be able to summon up and concentrate your willpower and attention on just one chosen task at a time. Once achieved, shift your focus to the next step in the journey. Try not to distract yourself by focusing on unrelated goals or goals you might tackle after you've done this one—just put your head down and do the task that's right in front of you. Then do the next.

Even as you take breaks, reassess your strategy, or take a moment to celebrate, you should still have in the back of your mind a good idea of where you are, where you're going, and what you need to do next. This keeps you motivated, focused, and on the path. After you've achieved a goal, you can be so busy celebrating that you open a little window for fresh excuses or distractions to come in. Don't give them a chance. Remember, as the old proverb goes, "there are mountains beyond the mountains." In other words, there is no goal that you can achieve that frees you completely from the need to know what your next move is. There are goals beyond goals.

- Try to work backward from your big goal, setting up smaller milestones. Monitor your progress on this path visually. For example, keep a weight chart visible in the bathroom or have markings on the side of your water bottle so you can see what percent of your goal you have reached so far

- Make your goals regular—daily goals can feed into bigger weekly ones, which then feed into monthly ones

- Make goals as small as possible while still feeling that they are moving you closer

- Check how you're doing and keep adjusting. It's far better to stick to a plan that you've had to scale down than to completely throw out a "perfect" plan that you nevertheless couldn't manage. If something doesn't work, *make* it work

- Never stop asking what is serving you and what isn't. Whether you fail to achieve your goal, achieve it, or even surpass it, take the opportunity to learn what you can from the experience. It's one thing being told what works, but another to gather your own evidence and know from experience what works

Tip 27: Share Your Story

Don't keep it a secret that you're exercising or eating better. Don't hide your achievements or experiences no matter how modest they may seem to you. Tell close friends and family so they can join in on your path. You'll achieve a few things at once by opening up to others:

- You'll get to enjoy a moment of pride and celebration, and share those good feelings with the people closest to you. If they've helped you along the way, this can also be a brilliant way of showing your appreciation and demonstrating that their faith in you was well founded!
- Knowing that you will in the future have achievements to share with others acts as a positive incentive, and essentially holds you accountable

- You'll combat any feelings of isolation or having to work on your dreams alone. Making big changes to your life can feel like lonely, secret work, but when you bring in the social element, you realize that you are not fighting your demons alone

- It may seem far-fetched now, but sharing your story can actually inspire and motivate others. You could set up a positive feedback loop where you are motivated to do well precisely because you know others are looking up to you and following your example. This in turn encourages them to be better, which then makes you feel good and determined to do the same yourself

- You will find it much easier to ask for help or support if the lines of communication are already open and people are fully on board with the changes you want to make

Are you one of those people who likes to hide the fact that you're on a diet? Maybe you do that thing where you turn down food by pretending to be allergic or lie about having eaten earlier. But consider that not being transparent actually makes it harder for you in the long run. It means that everything you do is down to you and you alone. People cannot support you, advise you, or celebrate with you if they don't know that you're trying to make the change in the first place. And without having witnesses along your path, it's much, much easier to quietly give up on yourself since nobody is looking and nobody (it feels like) cares.

Be honest and speak up. Tell people what you're going through. You might be surprised at the domino effect of good change that might start to fall around you if you make that step toward better health first. Inspire your family and close friends. It's not altruism—if everyone around you is also encouraged and positive, it will make it infinitely easier for you to do what you need to do.

- Share your goals, plans, and big ideas with others. Tell people what is inspiring and motivating you, and what dreams you have for yourself

- Also, share your challenges. Someone may relentlessly keep offering that enormous slice of cake when they think you're just being polite by turning it down, but they may understand if you pull them aside beforehand and explain what you're doing and why. Ask people outright for their support. Very few will be unwilling to give it if only you ask!

- Let people in on your schedule so they know where they stand with you. If you are communicating loud and clear that you do your YouTube workout every afternoon in the living room, there's a far greater chance you won't be interrupted

- Invite people to join you. Getting fit and healthy can be a very sociable thing. Can't decide whether to go for your afternoon run or see that friend who wants to visit? Do both by inviting them to come on a long hike with you instead. You'll strengthen

> your relationship and burn calories
> with no compromise on either side

Sharing openly and honestly with people can be a double-edged sword—we get more support and understanding, but in exchange, we have to give up some of our excuses. We can no longer sit secretly with our goals or quietly sabotage our plans because nobody would be any wiser. Stepping up and announcing loud and clear, "I am making a change, and I'm reaching out to others so you can join me," is an empowering act that will give you unexpected strength. Think of your support system as an offsite store of willpower!

Summary:

- The kinds of goals you set for yourself influence the likelihood of you achieving those goals. Make SMART goals—specific, measurable, attainable, realistic, and time-bound.
- Having goals helps you focus your intention, and celebrating when we reach them helps us keep track of

progress and make course corrections along the way.

- Setting realistic time frames for goals is a sign of self-respect and faith in your abilities. Make sure you have short-, medium-, and long-term goals in place.
- Don't fall into the trap of thinking that healthy living is boring and unpleasant. Splurge and reward yourself, but in healthy ways.
- Each time you reach a new milestone, take the time to update your self-image, feel proud of your achievement, and tell yourself that yes, you *are* a healthy, motivated, strong person.
- Your focus and commitment can slacken with time. Milestones are a great opportunity to reconnect to your goal and sharpen your focus.
- Finally, don't slog alone in secret. When you reach your milestones, no matter how small, rope in others to celebrate with you. Share your story, be honest, speak up about your challenges and your triumphs, and you may even find yourself in the position of inspiring and teaching others.

Epilogue

Speaking of celebrations and milestones reached, we've now arrived at the point in the book where congratulations are in order—you've finished the book, well done!

This is worth acknowledging. In reading this book, you have taken an important first step. You have sent the message to yourself that you are willing to make a change, that you are showing up to do the work, and now, in the final pages, you have proved to yourself that you can achieve (no matter how small that achievement might look!).

In each chapter, we've turned our attention to all the important ingredients necessary to make lasting, healthy changes to our lives. Good habits and routines, dedication, and a positive mindset are all essential building blocks.

To be successful, you ultimately need to be **pre-emptive** and **proactive**.

Take control. Make a plan and follow it consistently. Stay aware and never be afraid to try again, to readjust, or to go back to the drawing board completely. Constantly find realistic ways to bring your goals into real life by taking action. Be ruthless with yourself and expect a lot, but for all those times things don't go quite to plan, be ready and prepared to forgive yourself, have a little compassion, and quickly get on with your life.

Let's sum up the most important key points from the chapters above:

- Before you embark on a plan, summon sufficient dedication. This is a promise you make to yourself that you will commit to the sustained effort required to meet your goals, despite obstacles.

- Change is not an overnight miracle, but a long string of (boring) behaviors consistently repeated, i.e. habits. Work hard on your morning and evening routines and you pave the way for the day in between to be positive, prepared, and filled with focused energy.

- Your most important resource is your mindset. Without a conscious, positive frame of mind, you will always be undermining your hard work. Consider it a priority to regularly look within and determine whether your thoughts, attitudes, and core beliefs are really serving you—if not, change them.

- Expect bad days and prepare for them. It is always your responsibility to be honest about obstacles, to look at them clearly, and to find creative and realistic ways around them.

161

Knowing how to tap into your own source of inspiration is essential, as is learning to come to terms with the fact that change is uncomfortable.

- Finally, never forget that improving yourself should never feel like a slog. It is a privilege to be able to grow, to learn, and to be the best you can be. Enjoy it rather than constantly looking over the horizon to the reward or the day you can stop trying. Set deadlines, and when you reach those goals, celebrate and make sure to update the image you have of yourself as someone who can and does succeed. Stay focused and share your story—your new story of success—with those around you.

In the beginning of this book, I asked you a question: is real change possible? Hopefully, you have a slightly different answer now than when you began. Change is more than possible . . . for those who believe it to be so, and for those who are willing to put in the required effort.

Is that you?

Because action has been such a focus for us in this book, we're going to finish off with an exercise that you can do right now to condense the things you most want to take from each chapter. Below is a sample weekly plan. You don't need to replicate this in detail; rather, see how each of the tips covered has been applied, for maximum success. Following that is a summary sheet for you to extract those tips and ideas that are most likely to serve you at the stage of the path you're now on.

SAMPLE WEEKLY SCHEDULE

For the person using this schedule, the broad goal was as follows:

S – lose ten pounds in the coming month and/or an inch of the waistline
M – daily weigh-ins to see if weight has dropped, as well as body measurements
A – this is a moderate goal that is definitely achievable!

R – relevant to overall life goal of being healthier, feeling more confident, etc.

	Activity
Monday	• Lunch time walk – 3 miles • Do week's grocery shopping after work • 30 minute arm routine before dinner
Tuesday	• Hour-long ab and HIIT workout before dinner
Wednesday	• Lunch time walk – 3 miles
Thursday	• Hour-long lower body and HIIT workout before dinner
Friday	• Lunch time walk – 3 miles • Catch up with Marie and share progress stories
Saturday	• Big gym session with husband . . whether I like it or not :(• Therapy in the afternoon
Sunday	• Plan tomorrow's grocery shopping in detail • House tidy and laundry • Weekly weigh in and progress update. Goal adjustment • 1 hour yoga and flexibility training

T – will check in after a month

The above activities are combined each day with a morning and evening routine as follows:

Morning Routine:

6:30 – Wake up to gentle bird sounds alarm on other side of room. While in kitchen making coffee, do a few stretches, open curtains wide, and take a few deep breaths of morning air

6:45 – Drink coffee while sitting with a journal to plan the day ahead. Do a breathing meditation and positive visualization focusing on where I'm aiming for with my weight loss. Affirmations to tell myself I can do it. Make sure jogging shoes are ready and waiting in the kitchen—bring the mug to the dishwasher and be ready to go!

7:15 – Do a light jog around the block with the dog or an indoor workout if it's raining

8:00 – Hop in the shower, get ready and dressed. Vitamins. Floss.

8:30 – Feed dog and eat the pre-prepared oats from night before. Grab a banana for the road. Run a quick checklist to see I have everything I need for the day.

9:00 – Leave for work. Listen to pre-selected inspirational podcast on the way. Eat banana. Be grateful for banana. Park at work, take a deep breath, gather myself, and start the workday like a boss.

Evening routine:

6:00 – Hour exercise, or if it's a rest day, a little housework or shopping

7:00 – Make and eat pre-planned dinner, then clean up kitchen. A square of fancy dark chocolate for dessert if I want, and some herbal tea.

8:00 – Prepare tomorrow's oats, make sure I have a clean and ironed outfit ready, set any alarms, put my water bottle in the fridge. Feed dog.

8:15 – Settle down for either an hour of TV, reading, or a hobby. No more than one hour of TV, though! Could go for a stroll after dinner if the weather's nice.

9:15 – Meditate and journal. Listen to music. Quiet time with family or husband, fancy bath if it's cold. A little prayer and refresh my commitment to take the very best care of my body that I can
10:15 – Read in bed a little till drowsy
10:30 – Lights out and sleep

Now, it's over to you. You've read this book, now do yourself the favor of not forgetting anything of value that you might be able to take from it (granted, some people will take more, some less). The following sheet can help you capture and keep what matters most to you.

My SMART goal and why it matters to me (written as a promise or commitment to yourself)	
Weak spots in my current lifestyle and how I can address them	
3 things I'd like to introduce into my morning routine, starting tomorrow	
3 things I'd like to introduce into my evening routine, starting tomorrow	
How I can break down my main goal into monthly, weekly, and daily milestones	
1 thing I know I can do right now to prepare myself for inevitable setbacks	
How I want to picture myself at the end of this process, celebrating. How I want my image to change	
The single biggest lesson I want to take from reading this book, PLUS ONE WAY I CAN TURN THIS LESSON INTO CONCRETE ACTION	

Remember, change is possible for those who believe it and those who are willing to put in the work. You can be that person, not just starting from tomorrow, but *right now*. It's a choice. A choice you refresh and renew every week, every day, even every second. There are many people who have gone before you, and you can take guidance and strength from them. In the same way, know that there are many other people coming after you, and the choices you make right now have the potential to inspire and lead them on the same path . . . if you make it so. Good luck!

Summary Guide

- There is no optimal way to start your morning—the best morning routine is one that fits with *your* personal values, limitations, and goals.
- With a morning routine, you take charge of the day and steer it in the direction you want it to go. Start with one or two tweaks first, rather than changing everything all at once.
- Plan your morning the day before and draw up a detailed schedule.
- Even if you don't have a full workout, engage in some form of physical movement to wake up your body. Try stretching, deep breathing, walking, or yoga.
- If you do a morning workout, take your time to warm up properly. Morning workouts can set your day up for success.

- You don't have to eat breakfast—fasting in the morning can have incredible health and weight loss benefits. If you choose to have breakfast, though, plan it the night before and go for something small, protein-packed, and convenient.

- Finally, don't rush in the mornings. A solid plan and enough time will ensure you move through your morning routine without chaos or stress. Deliberately factor in quiet time where you journal, plan the day ahead, contemplate, meditate, or simply enjoy breakfast or coffee outside while orienting to the day ahead.

CHAPTER 2: DEDICATION

- Dedication is about making a promise to yourself to systematically rework old habits and thought patterns and replace them with better, healthier ones. Dedication means committing to following through with your goals, regardless of the obstacles in the way.

- Dedication matters because change is uncomfortable, and it takes energy and focus to shift us out of our status quo. Dedication helps us feel confident in our ability to do better, and fortifies our willpower.
- Being more dedicated is about taking your goals and bringing them to life by *taking concrete action*. Break goals down into small steps and act toward them every day.
- Remember that baby steps are more effective than quantum leaps. Make the smallest sustainable change possible, not the biggest change, since this is what adds up to big rewards in the long run.
- To start making progress and gaining momentum, begin with the "lowest hanging fruit." Identify your weak spots first and take action to replace those bad habits. This will give you the highest return on your efforts and motivate you to keep going.
- It can be especially tough to develop healthy habits in the workplace, so make sure you have a plan in place for how to keep your dedication going at work. If

something's not working, ask, "How can I *make* this work?"

<u>CHAPTER 3: FOCUS AND MENTALITY</u>

- When making improvements to your life, your focused and positive mindset is one of your greatest assets. Rather than being blindly "positive," you can simply become aware of where your focus and attention are going, and what you're choosing to create for yourself. Focus on solutions, not problems. Make it work.

- Regular milestones are necessary to keep up your motivation and focus. Schedule mini-milestones or rewards daily, weekly, and monthly. Take the time to acknowledge progress.

- When rewarding yourself, do so in a way that doesn't undermine your progress. Remember that you're celebrating your better self, and rewards should help you enjoy your healthier life, not pull you back to your old, unhealthy life.

- *All* diet philosophies have some value— what makes them work is your positive mindset, your dedication, and your consistent action. Whatever diet you choose, it will succeed if you practice some form of control, and if you're mindful of your consumption.

- Willpower and energy are finite. To preserve them, automate certain choices so it's easy to automatically make the right choice and harder to make the wrong one.
- Piece together a personal healthy living manifesto of rules that help you decide how to act. This helps you set boundaries, banish excuses, and turn down temptation.

CHAPTER 4: NIGHT ROUTINE

- A night routine consolidates and closes off the day, giving you time to check in on yourself and prepare for the next day. Your night routine influences the quality of your sleep that night, which in turn influences the following day. Thus, night routines and morning routines go hand

174

in hand to create a structured, productive, and healthy lifestyle.

- At night, focus on winding down, relaxing, and coming to an awareness of yourself and what's happened throughout the day. As with morning routines, make a small change, give it time, observe and tweak, then make another small change.

- Make your most impactful changes first. For most people, this means going to bed earlier and getting more (and better quality) sleep. Start with sleeping at the same time every night and see if there are any weak spots in your sleep hygiene.

- After a day of activity, pull back and enjoy quiet, gentle time alone. Reflect, journal, appraise the day past, and let things settle and digest.

- Plan the day ahead so you are ready to go first thing in the morning. It's easier to relax into deep sleep when you are confident that you're prepared to face the new day.

- Take a moment to remind yourself of why you're changing, and see how far you've come on your journey. Renew your commitment to yourself, refresh your willpower, and give yourself a pat on the back for all you've achieved.

CHAPTER 5: OVERCOMING BAD DAYS

- Change is always possible, but obstacles, setbacks, and failure are a given. To make successful changes, you need to anticipate and prepare for these setbacks.
- Be mindful of when you feel like giving up, and try to act as early as possible to adjust, take a rest, or find a creative way around the problem. If you mess up, the key is to ask what you can learn from the mistake, then immediately commit to action that puts you back on the path again. Forgive yourself and move on, empowered to do better next time.
- If you're getting impatient or demoralized, you may need to have more frequent milestones or rewards, or else re-evaluate your expectations.

- On bad days, instead of giving up, try to mix things up instead. Novelty and creativity can get momentum going again.
- Make sure you know where to find a renewable source of inspiration; tap into motivational quotes, podcasts, books, etc. to keep you inspired.
- Don't go it alone—find accountability with others.
- If you're having a very hard time, it may be worth having a closer look at your mindset, your core beliefs, your expectations, or the way you're framing your goals. Remind yourself that change is possible—your job is simply to find out how it's possible.
- Finally, make friends with discomfort and uncertainty. Getting out of your comfort zone is hard, but it's where change happens!

CHAPTER 6: REACHING MILESTONES

- The kinds of goals you set for yourself influence the likelihood of you achieving those goals. Make SMART goals—specific, measurable, attainable, realistic, and time-bound.

- Having goals helps you focus your intention, and celebrating when we reach them helps us keep track of progress and make course corrections along the way.

- Setting realistic time frames for goals is a sign of self-respect and faith in your abilities. Make sure you have short-, medium-, and long-term goals in place.

- Don't fall into the trap of thinking that healthy living is boring and unpleasant. Splurge and reward yourself, but in healthy ways.

- Each time you reach a new milestone, take the time to update your self-image, feel proud of your achievement, and tell yourself that yes, you *are* a healthy, motivated, strong person.

- Your focus and commitment can slacken with time. Milestones are a great opportunity to reconnect to your goal and sharpen your focus.

- Finally, don't slog alone in secret. When you reach your milestones, no matter how small, rope in others to celebrate with you. Share your story, be honest, speak up about your challenges and your triumphs, and you may even find yourself in the position of inspiring and teaching others.

www.ingramcontent.com/pod-product-compliance
Lightning Source LLC
Chambersburg PA
CBHW010246030426
42336CB00022B/3321